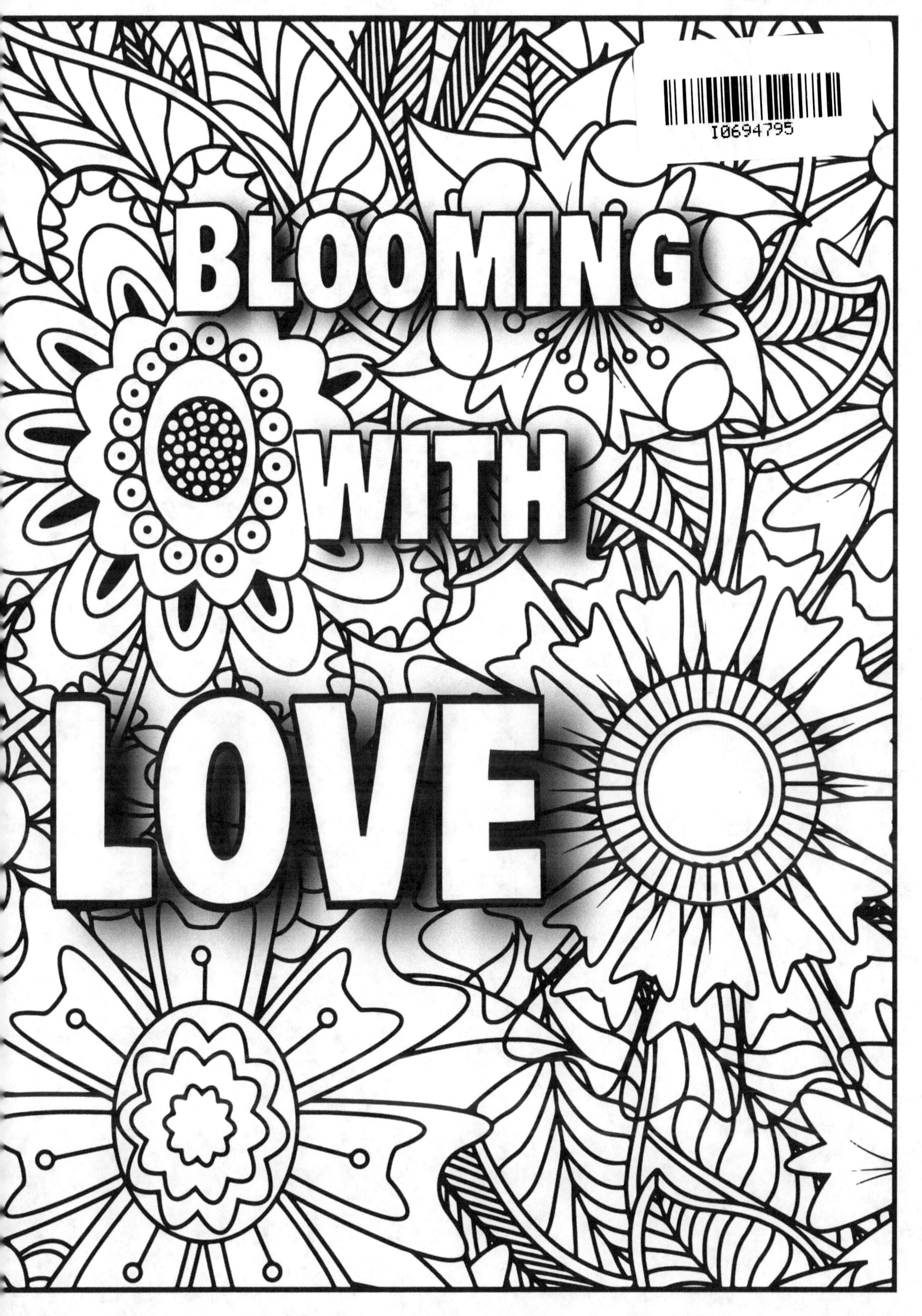

BLOOMING
WITH
LOVE

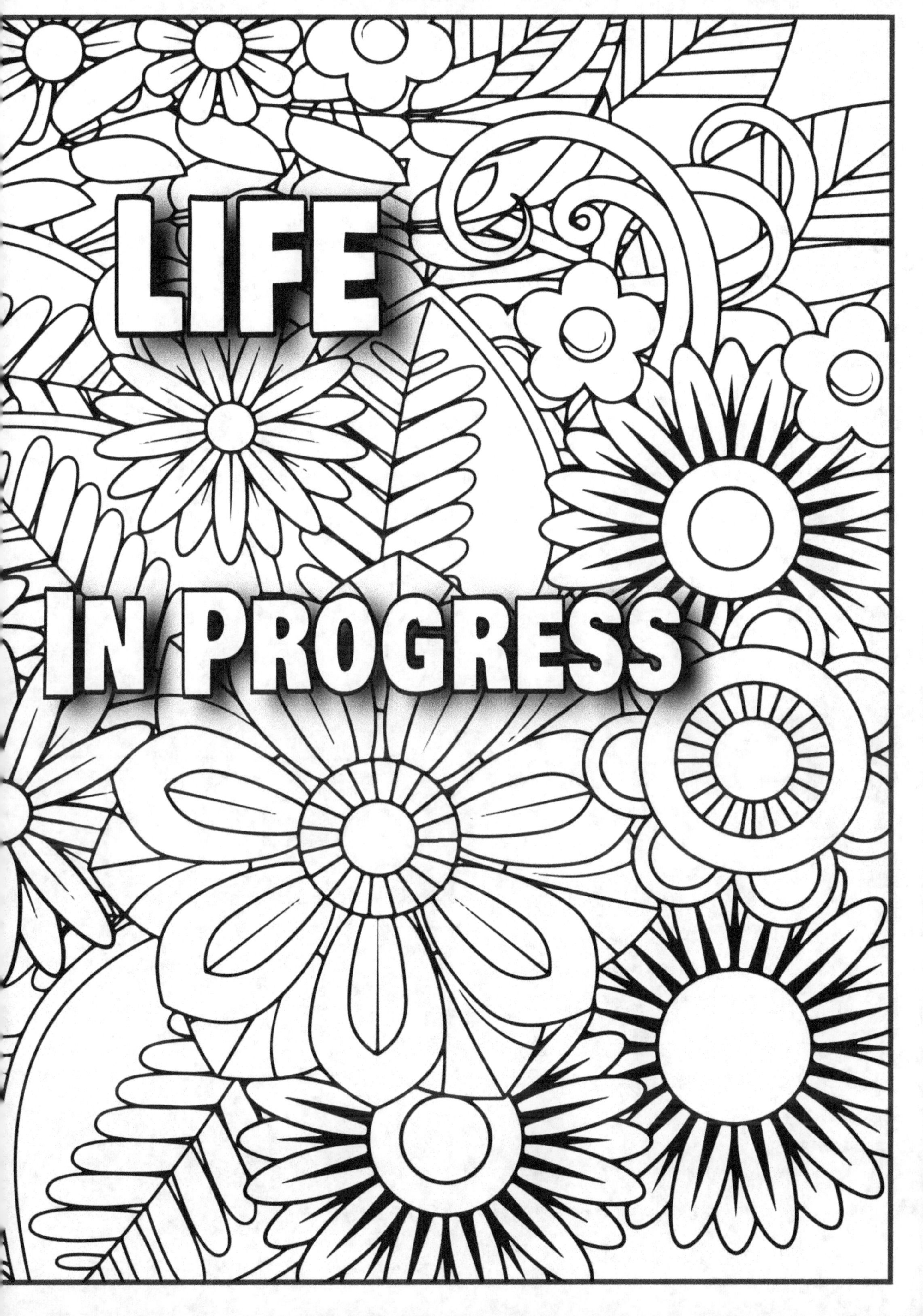

LIFE
IN PROGRESS

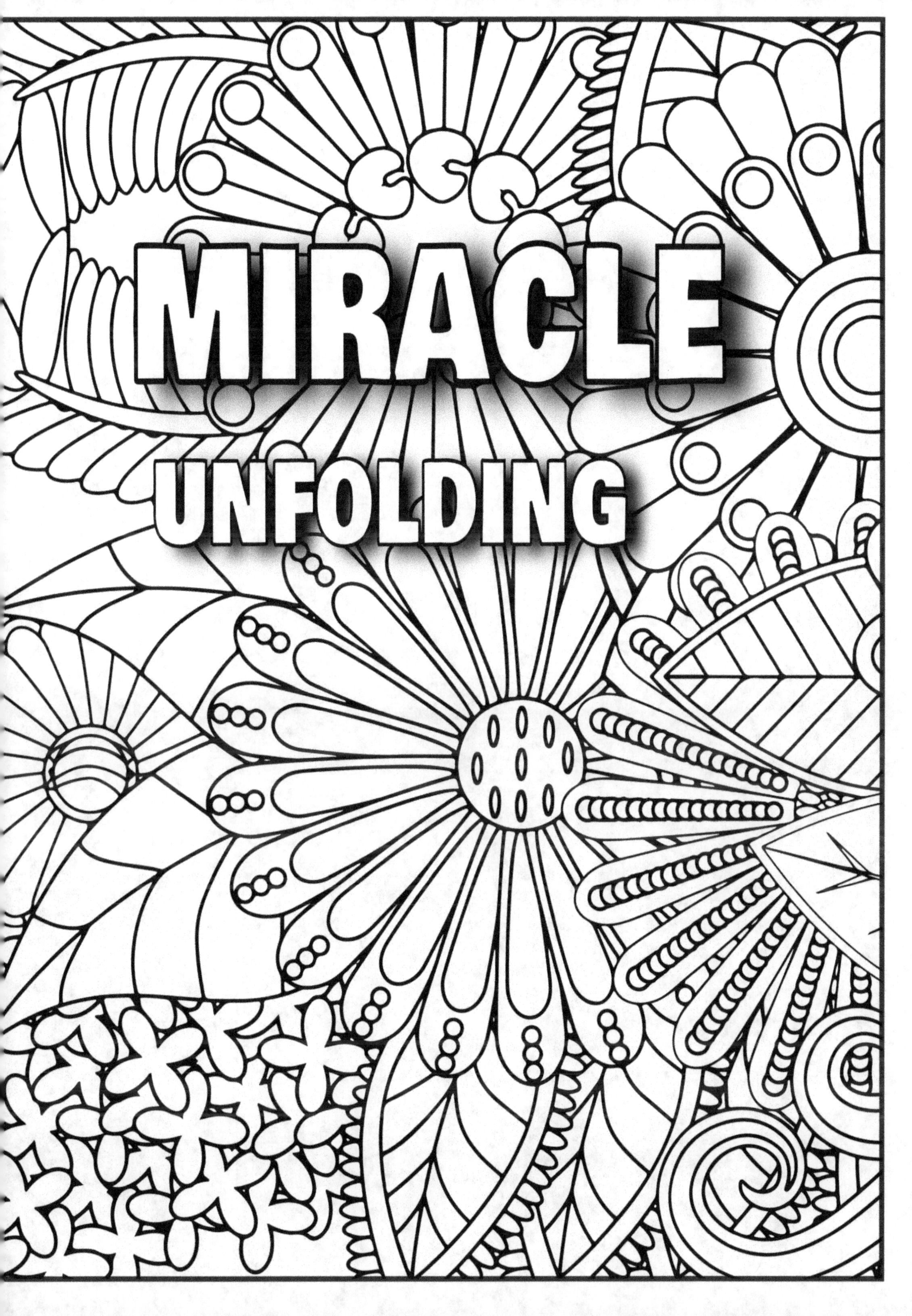

MIRACLE
UNFOLDING

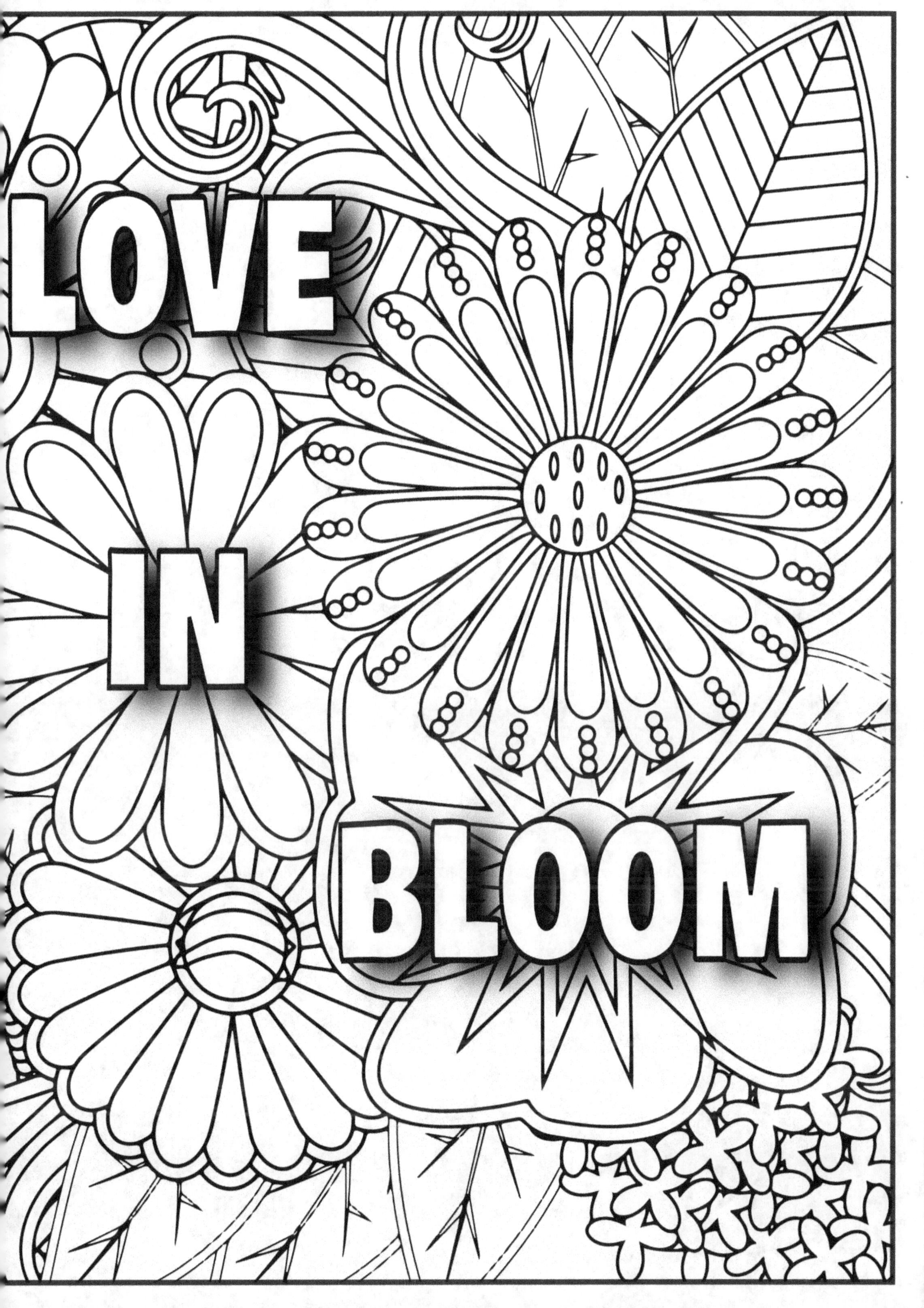

LOVE
IN
BLOOM

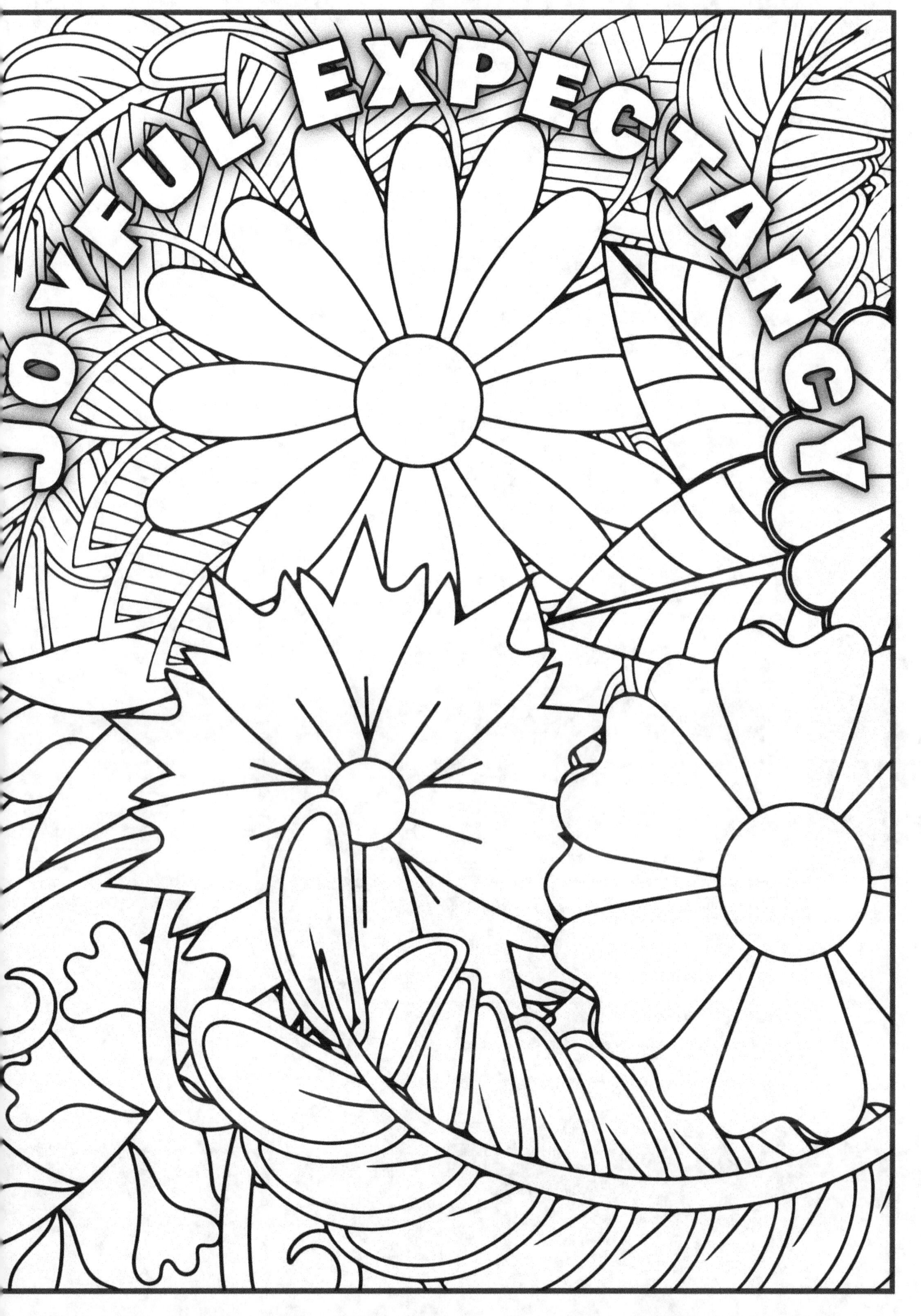

JOYFUL EXPECTANCY

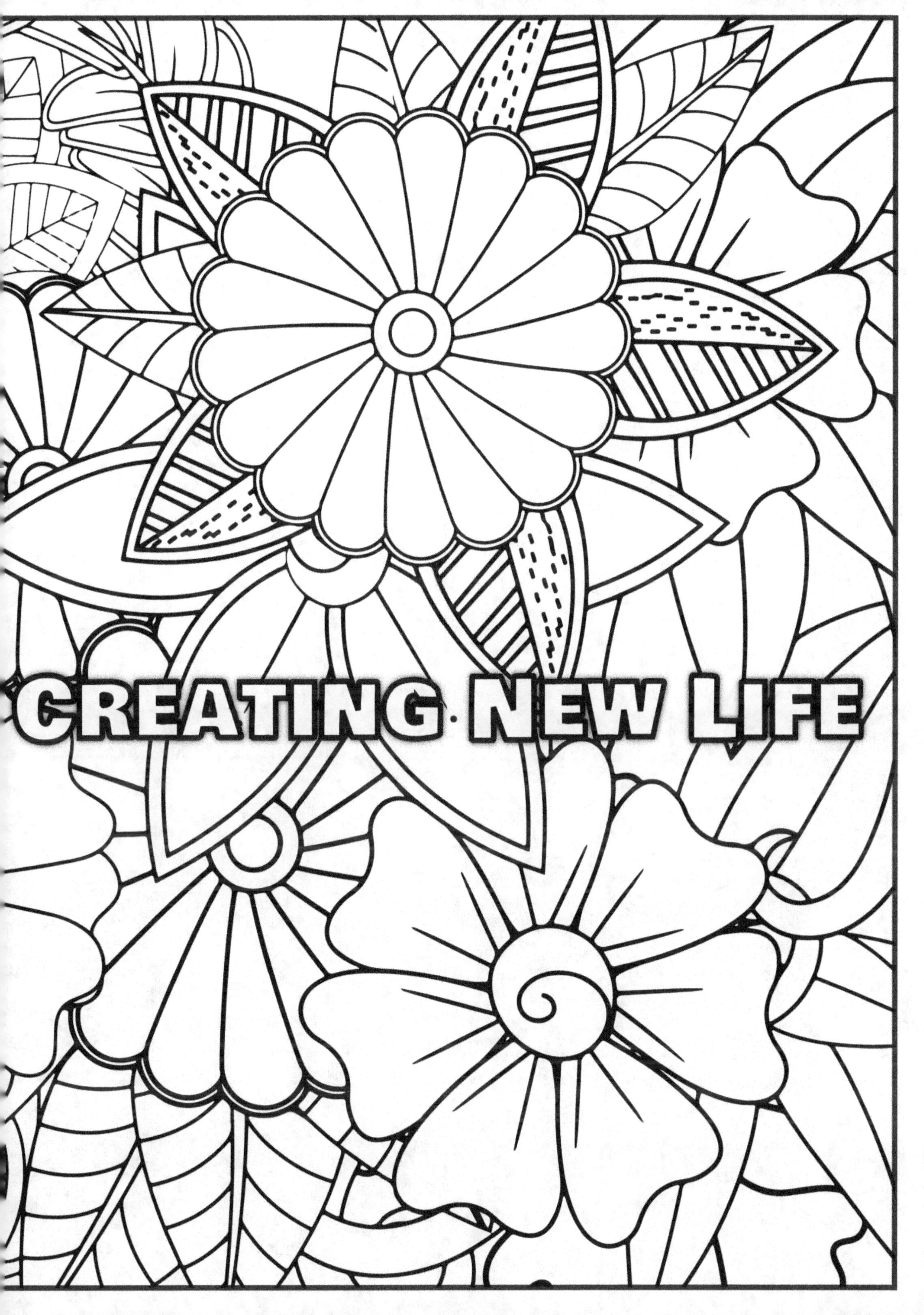
CREATING NEW LIFE

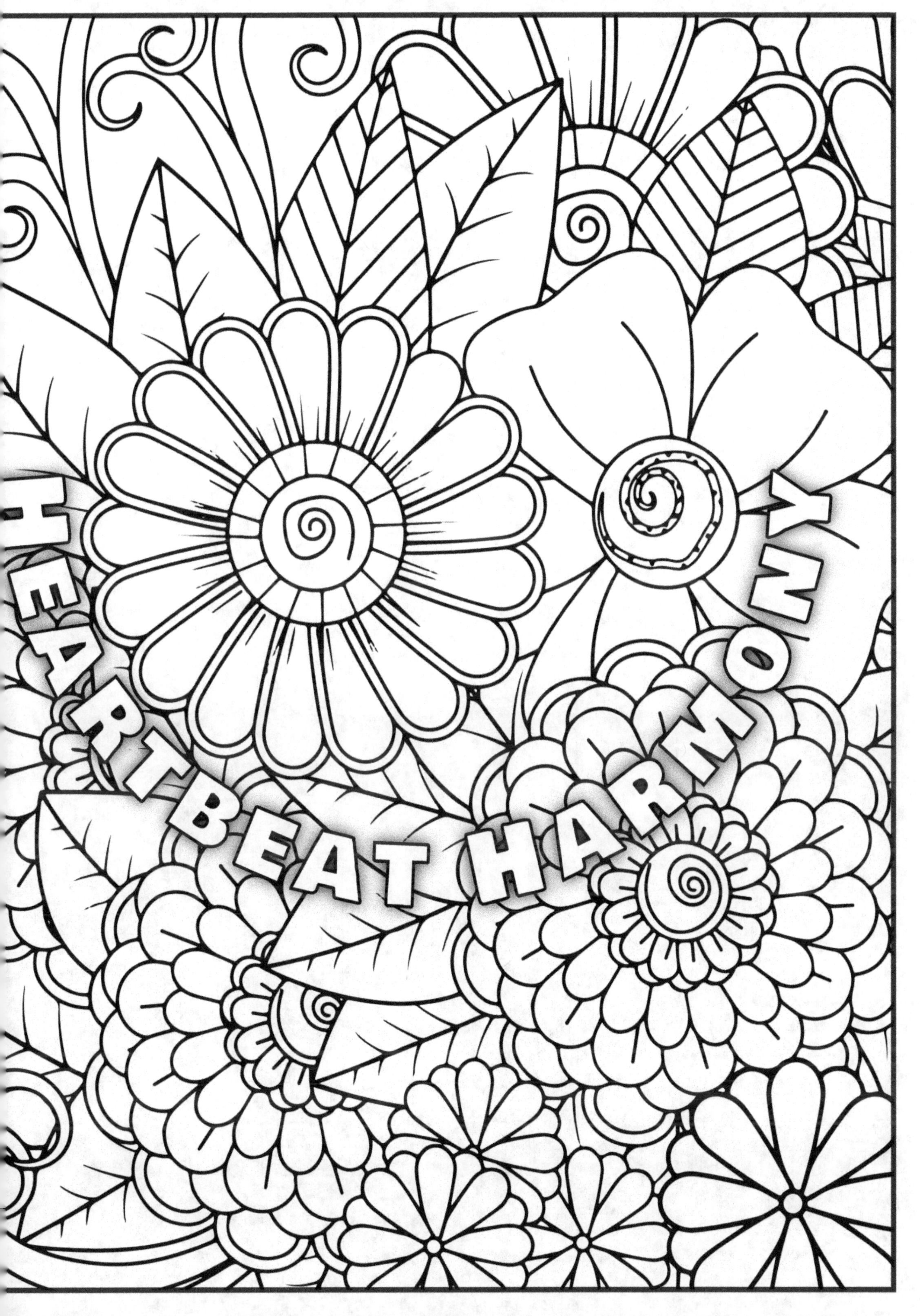

HEARTBEAT HARMONY

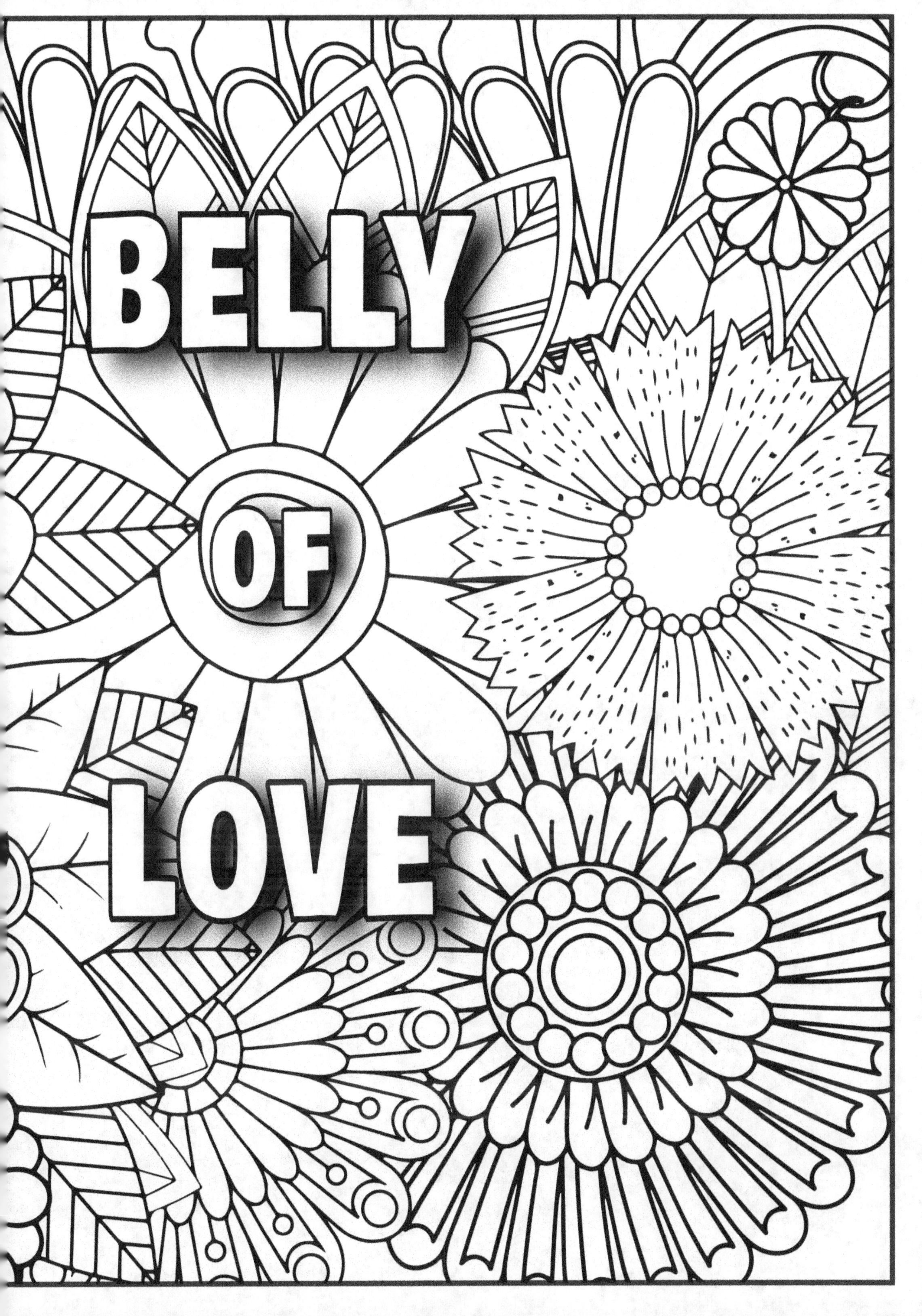

BELLY
OF
LOVE

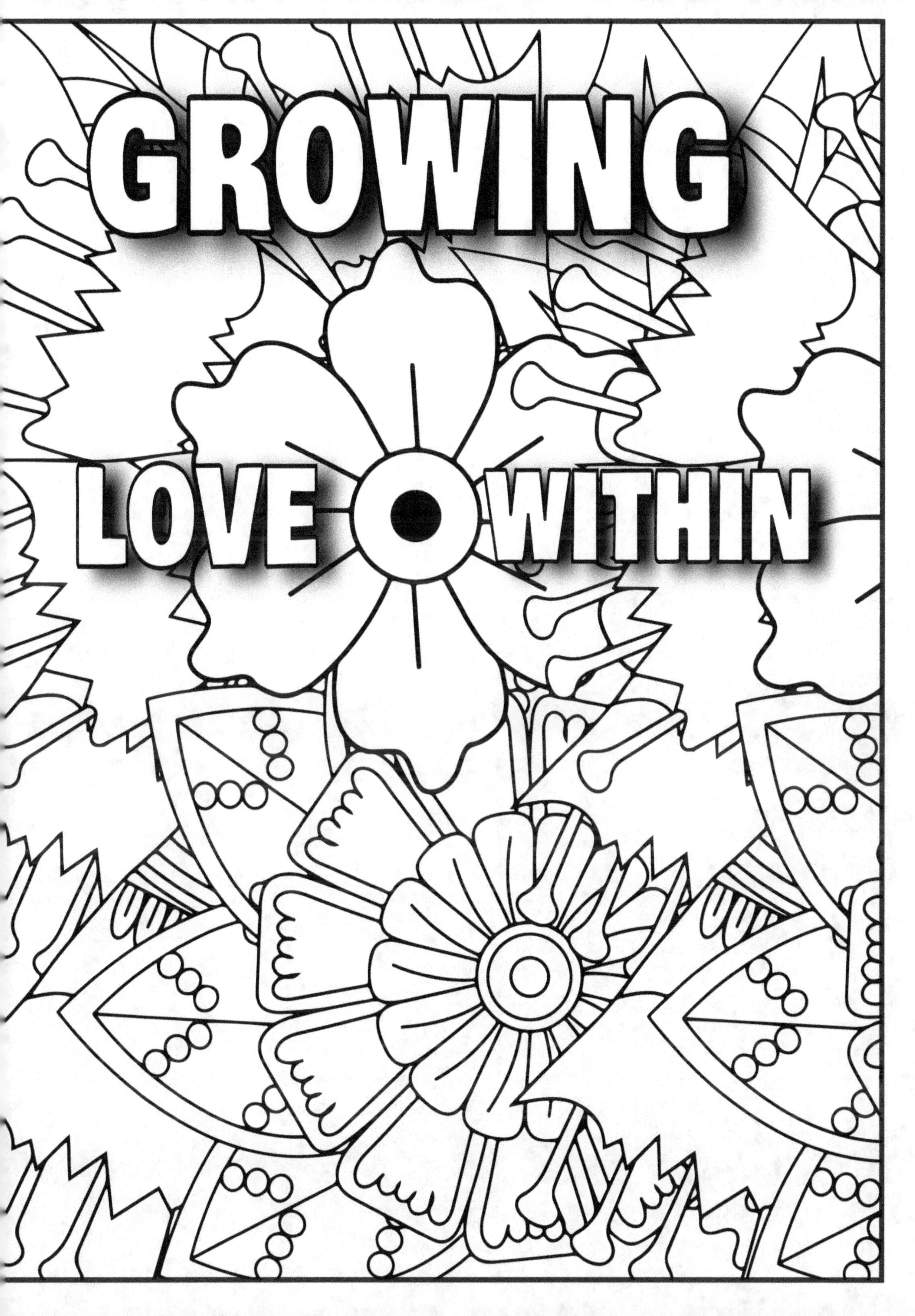

GROWING
LOVE
WITHIN

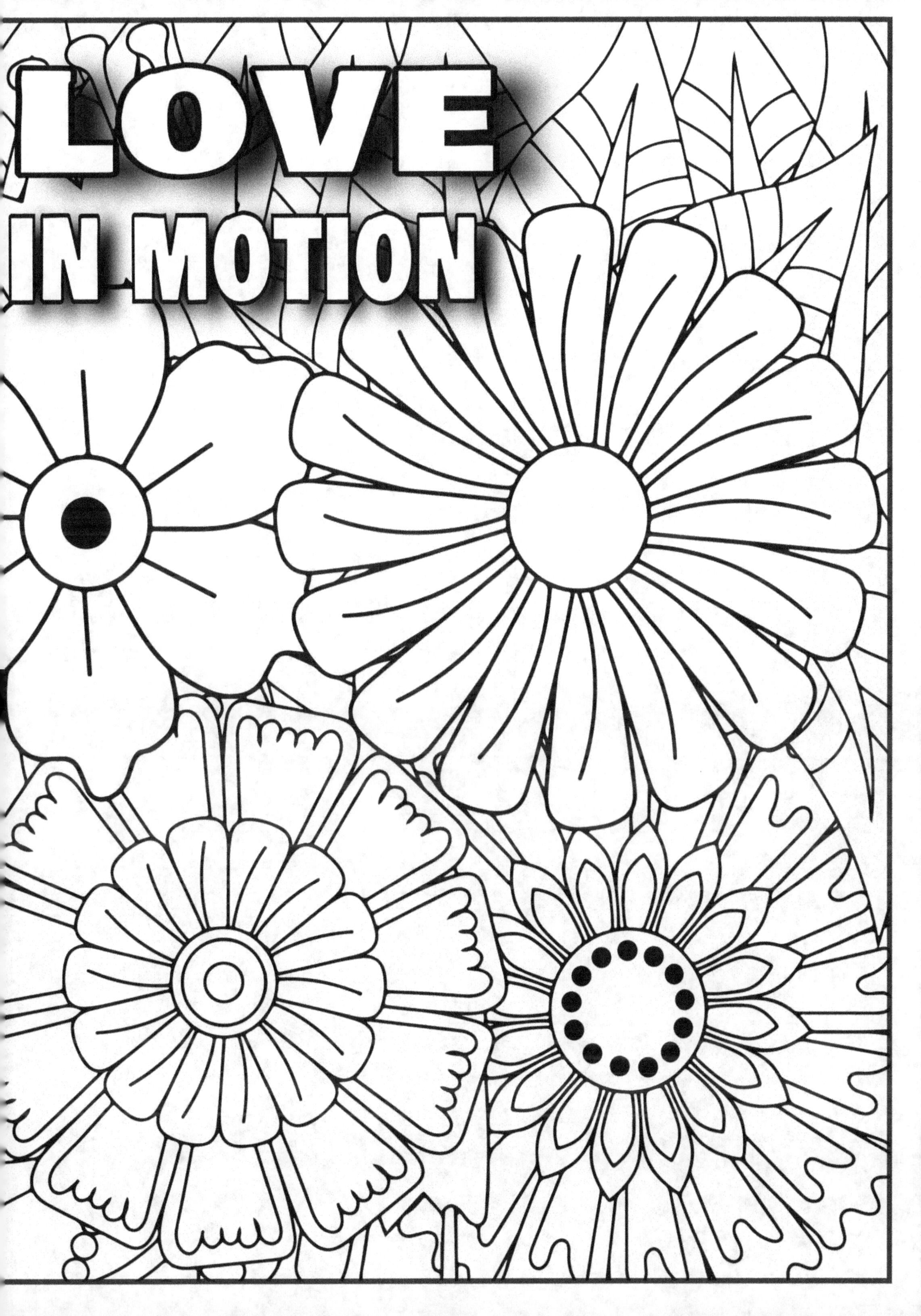

LOVE
IN MOTION

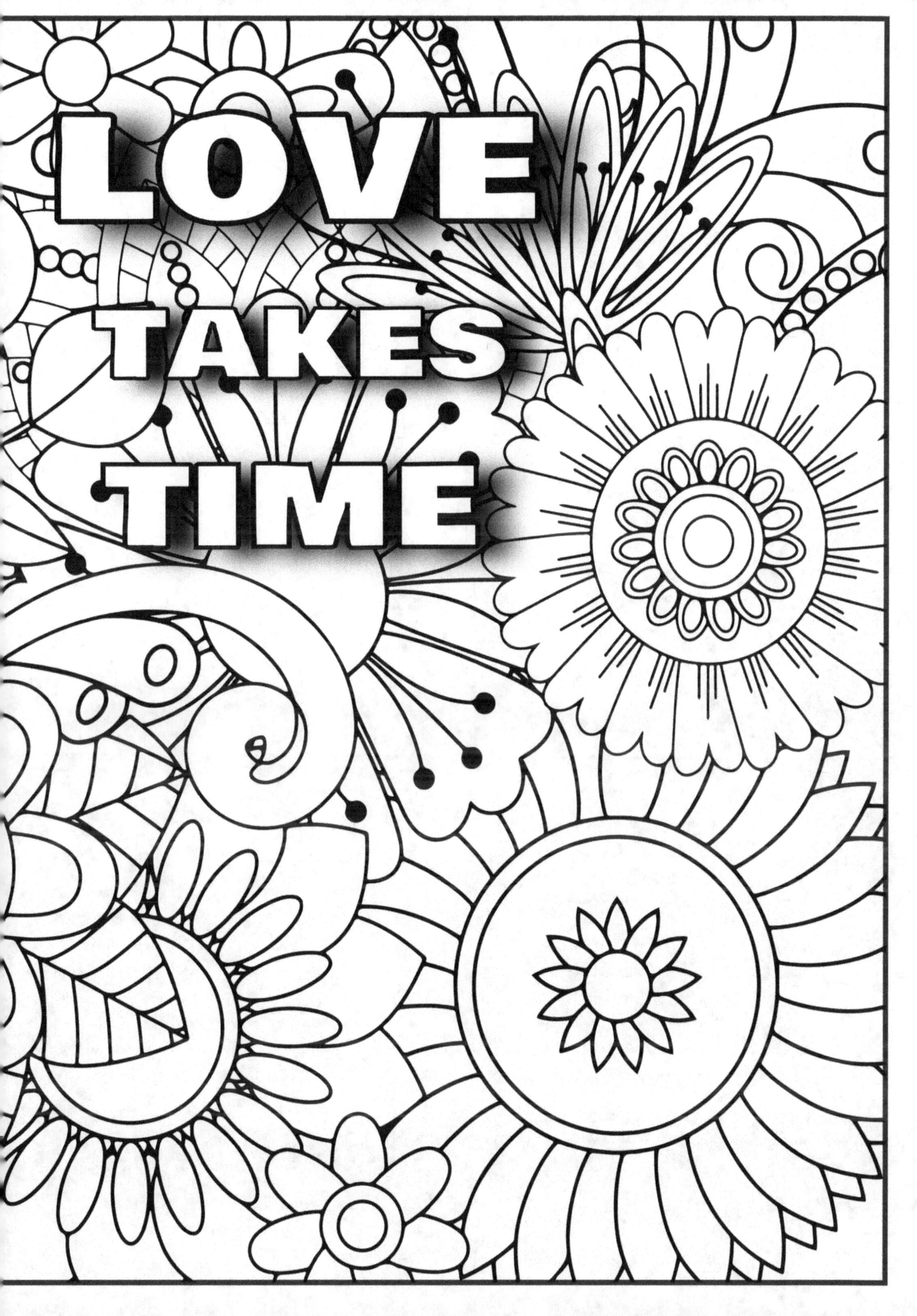

LOVE
TAKES
TIME

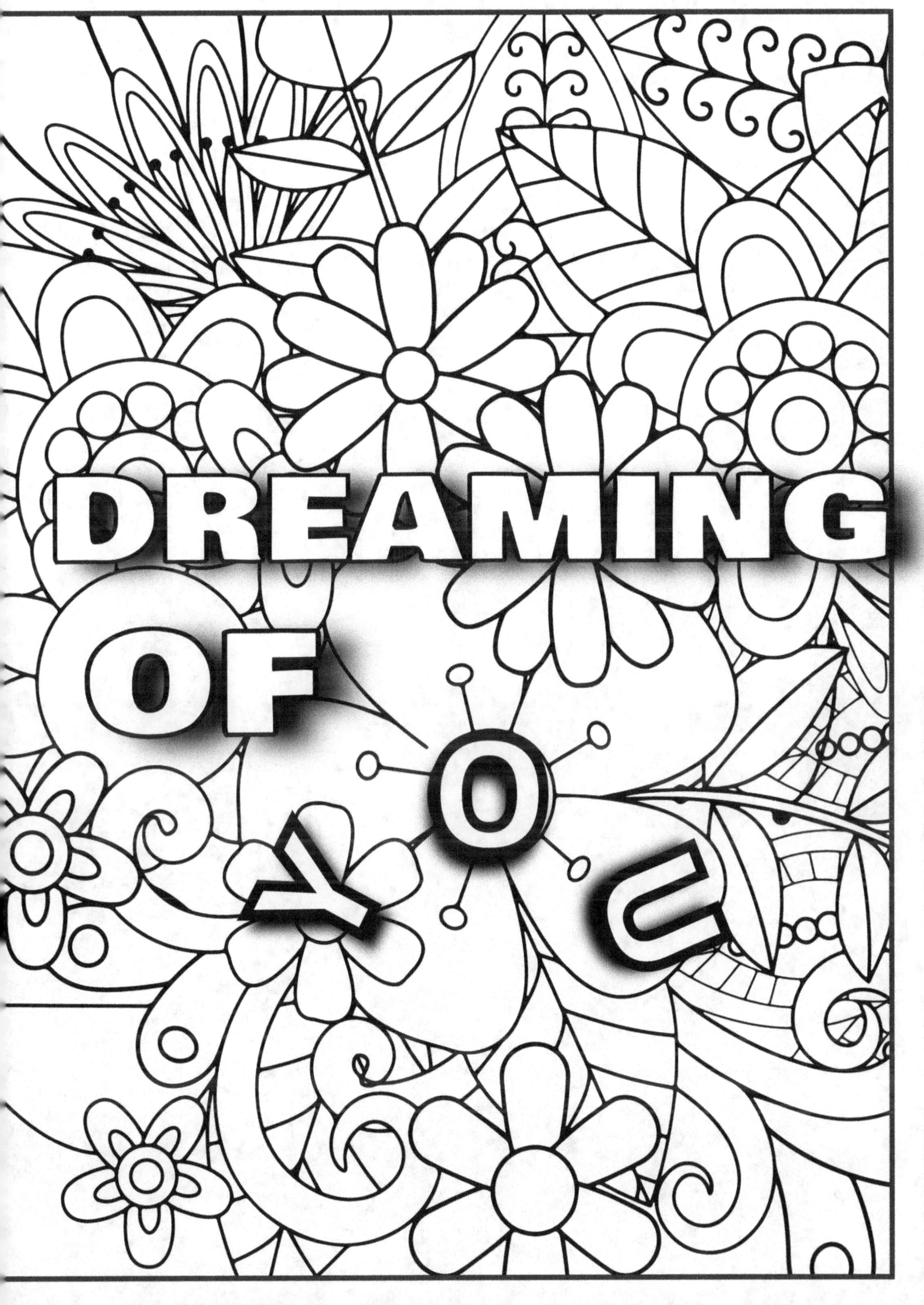

DREAMING
OF
YOU

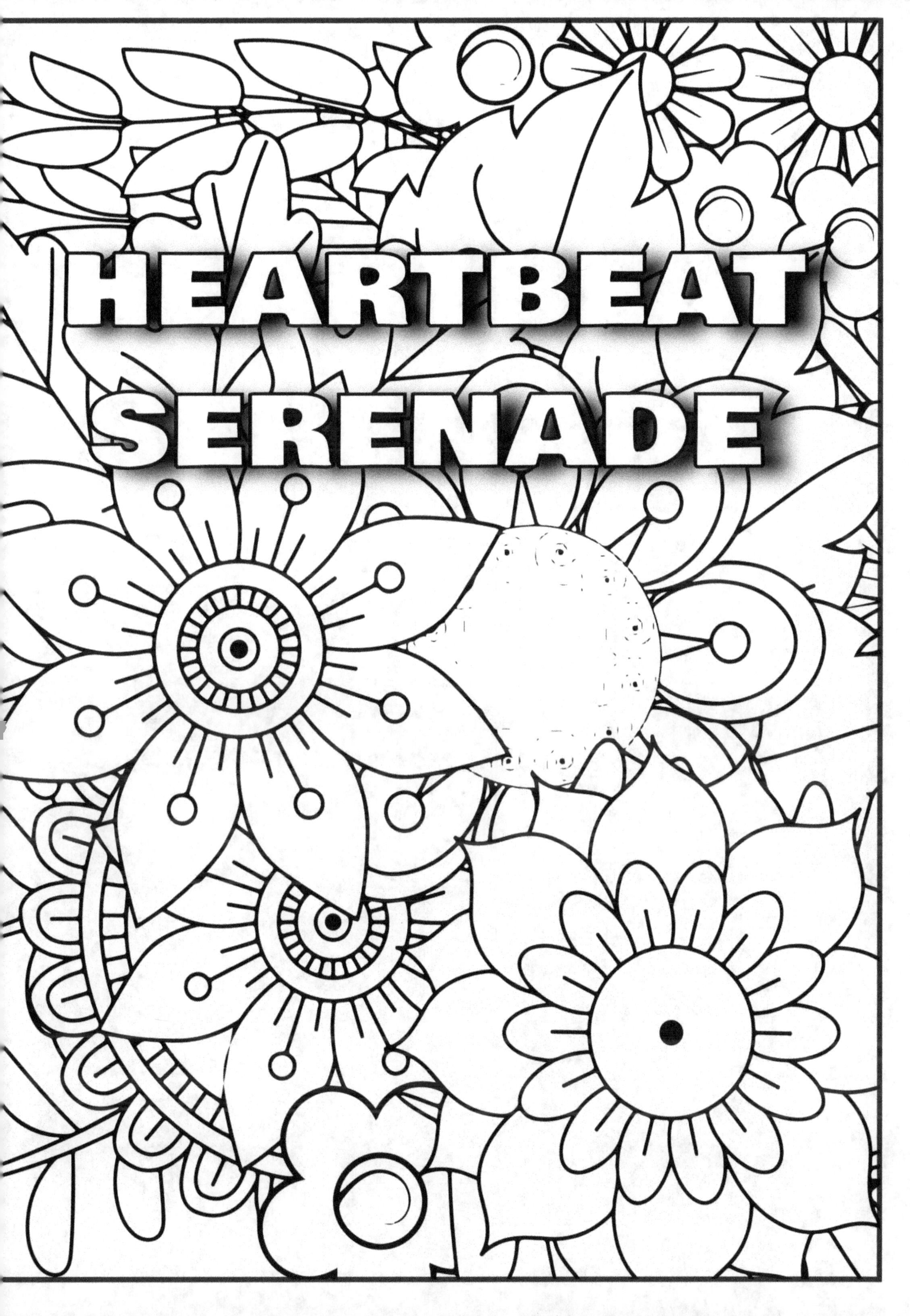
HEARTBEAT
SERENADE

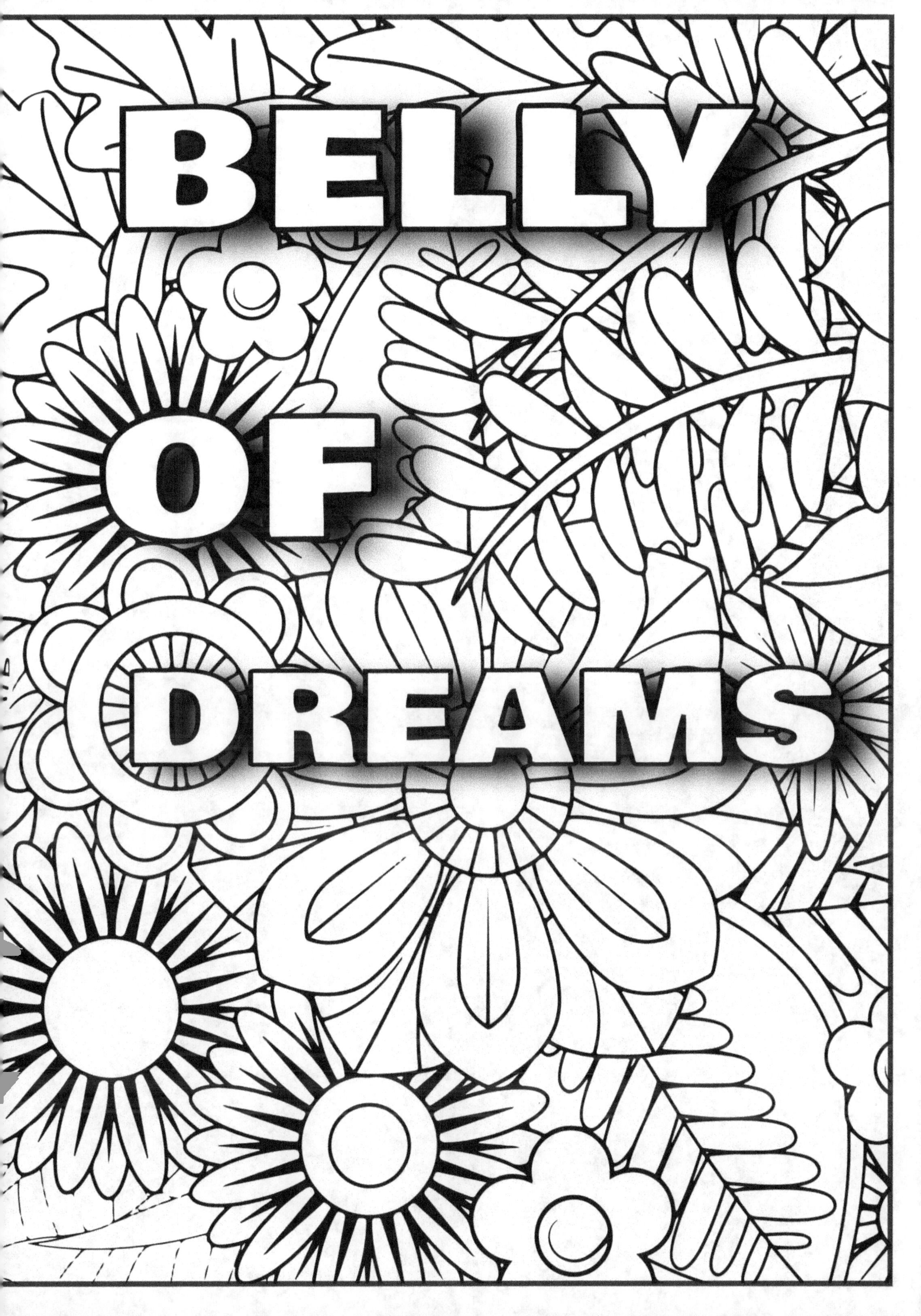

BELLY
OF
DREAMS

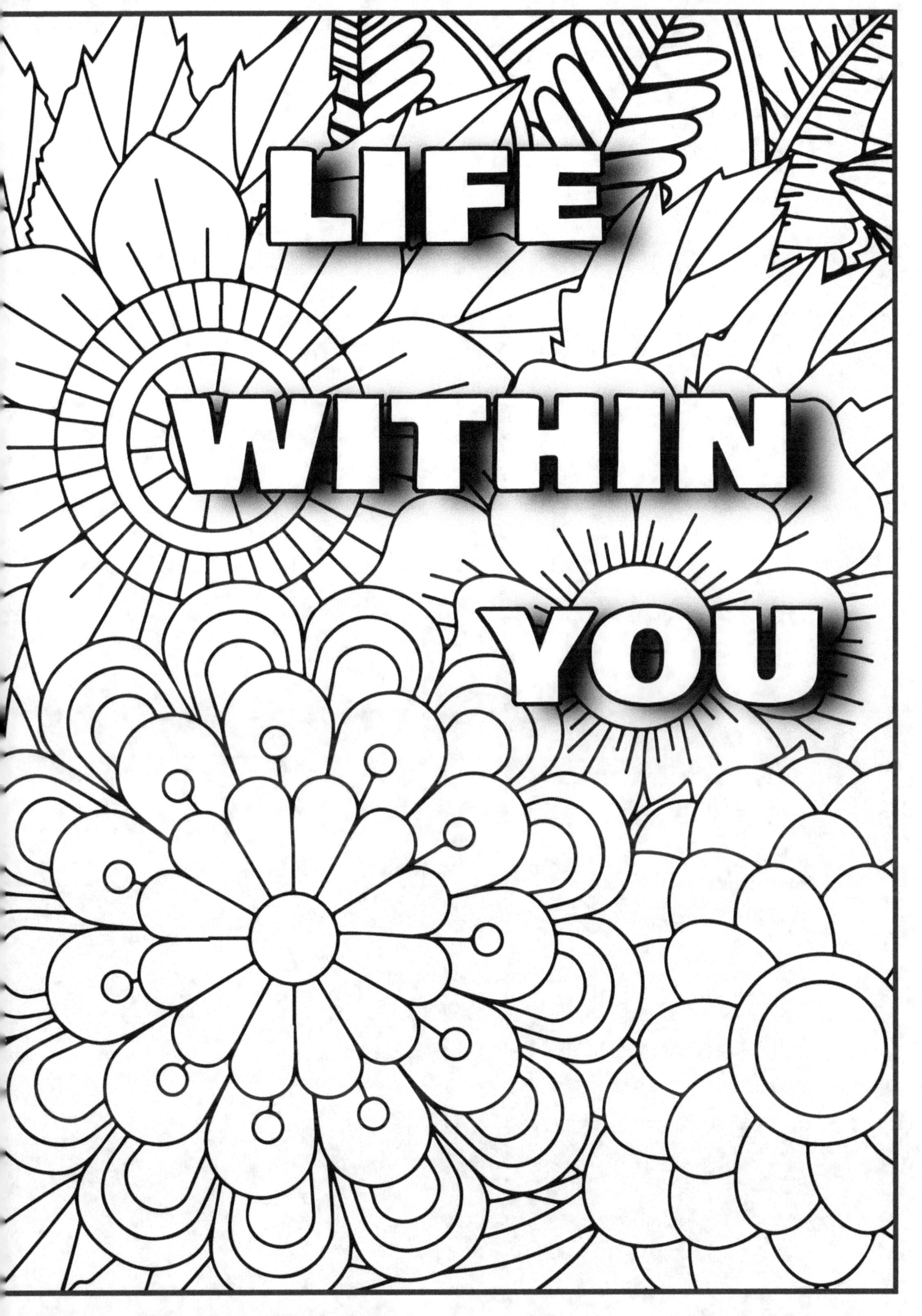

LIFE
WITHIN
YOU

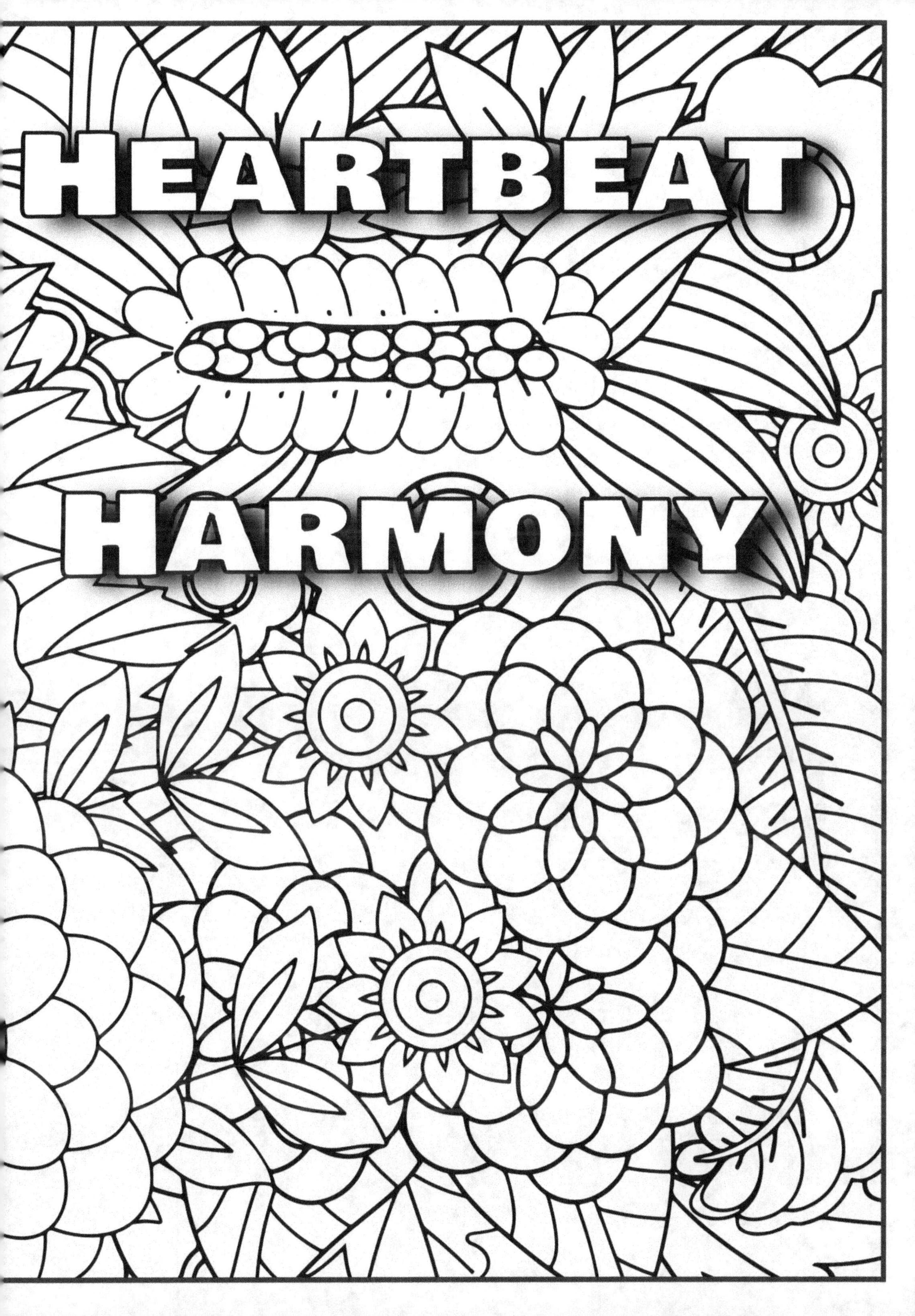

HEARTBEAT
HARMONY

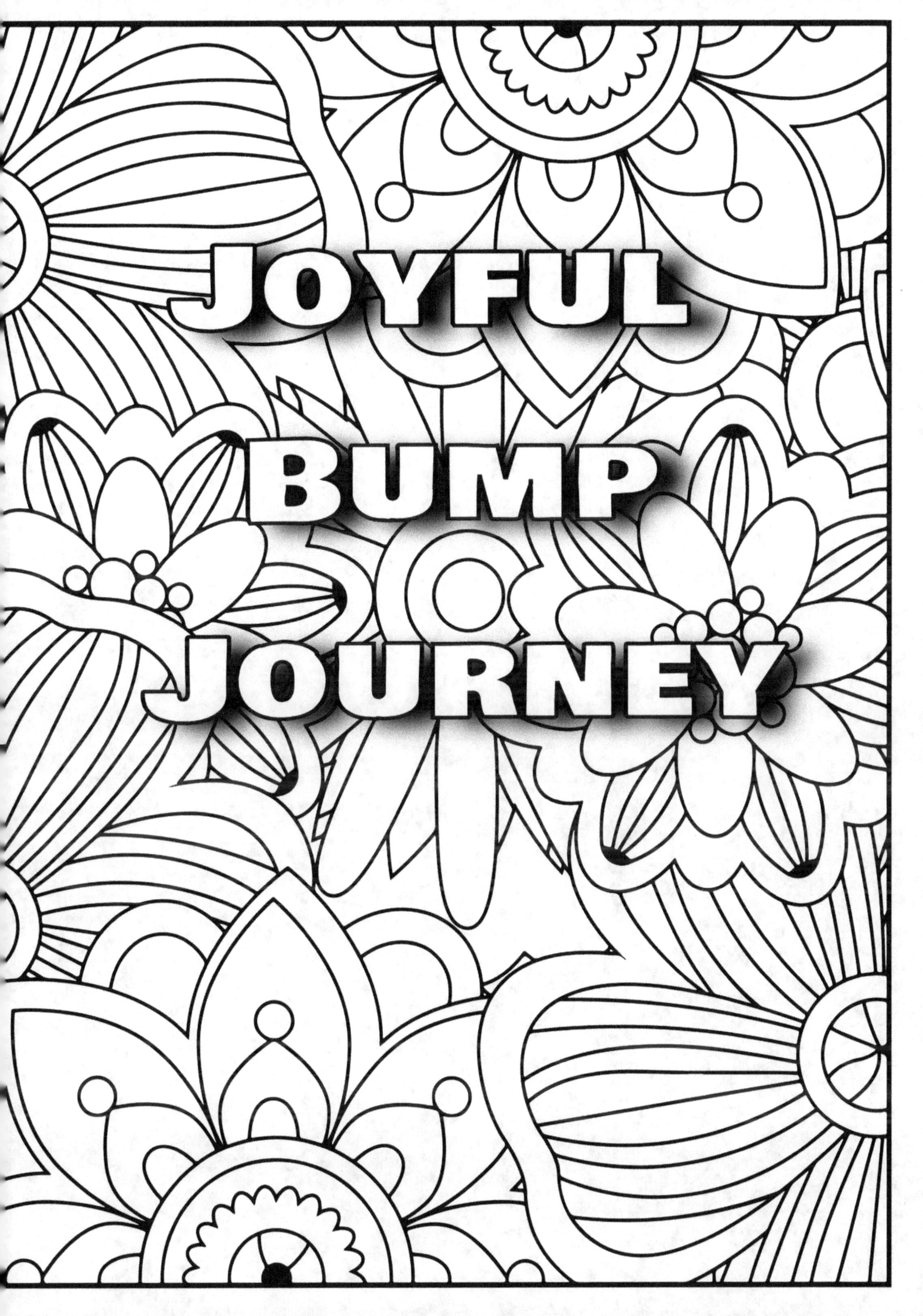

JOYFUL
BUMP
JOURNEY

GROWING JOY INSIDE

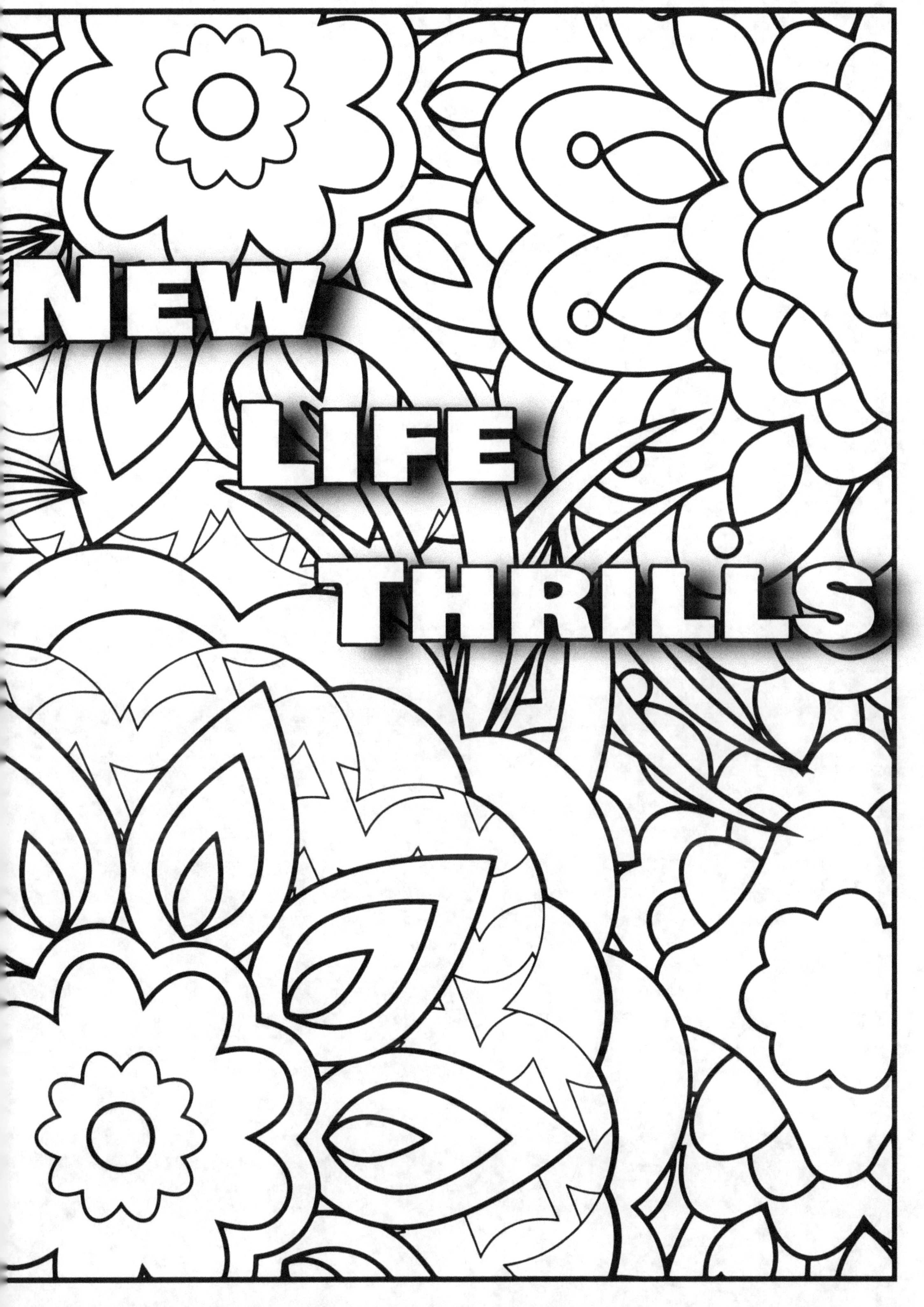

NEW
LIFE
THRILLS

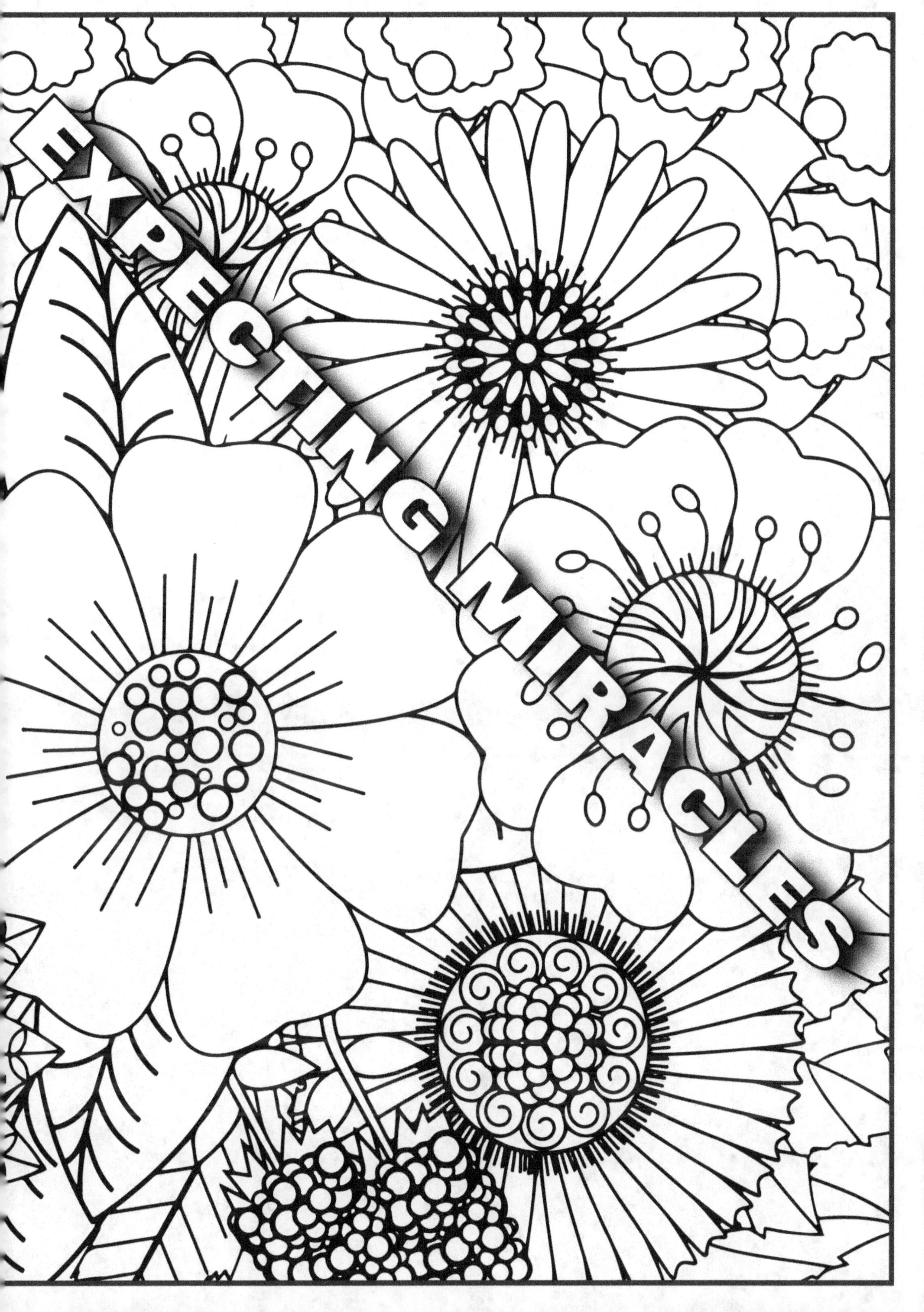

EXPECTING MIRACLES

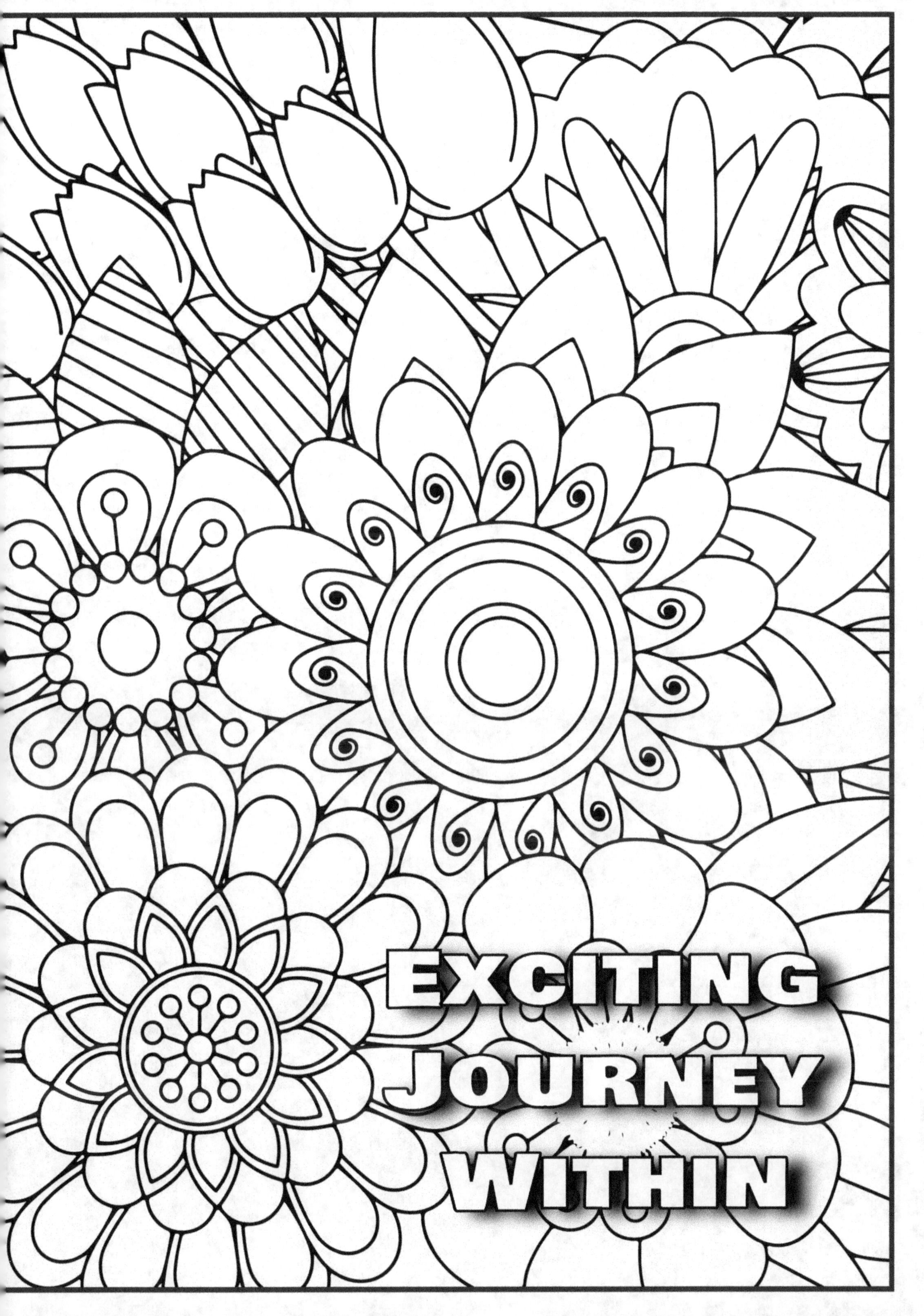
EXCITING
JOURNEY
WITHIN

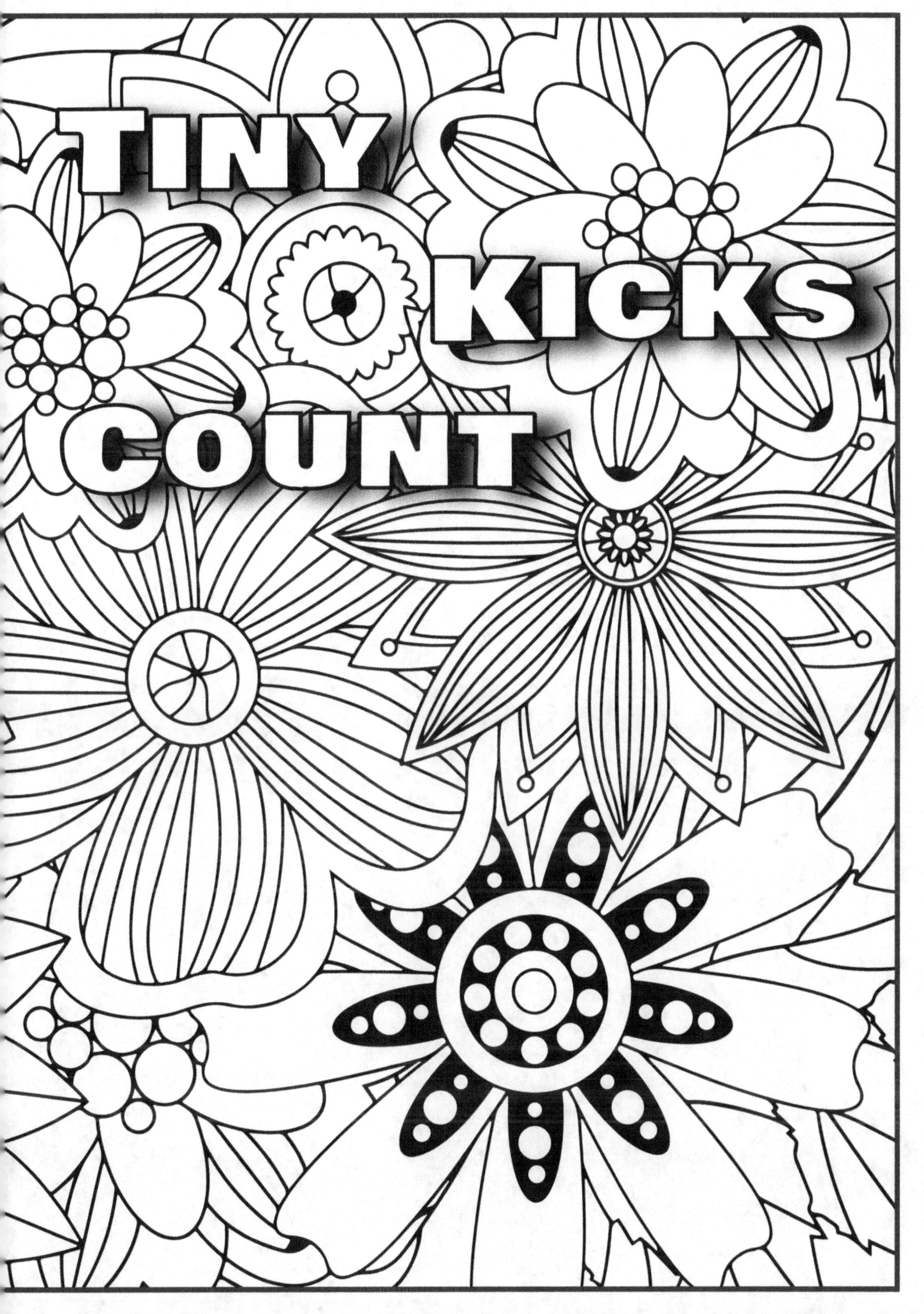

TINY
KICKS
COUNT

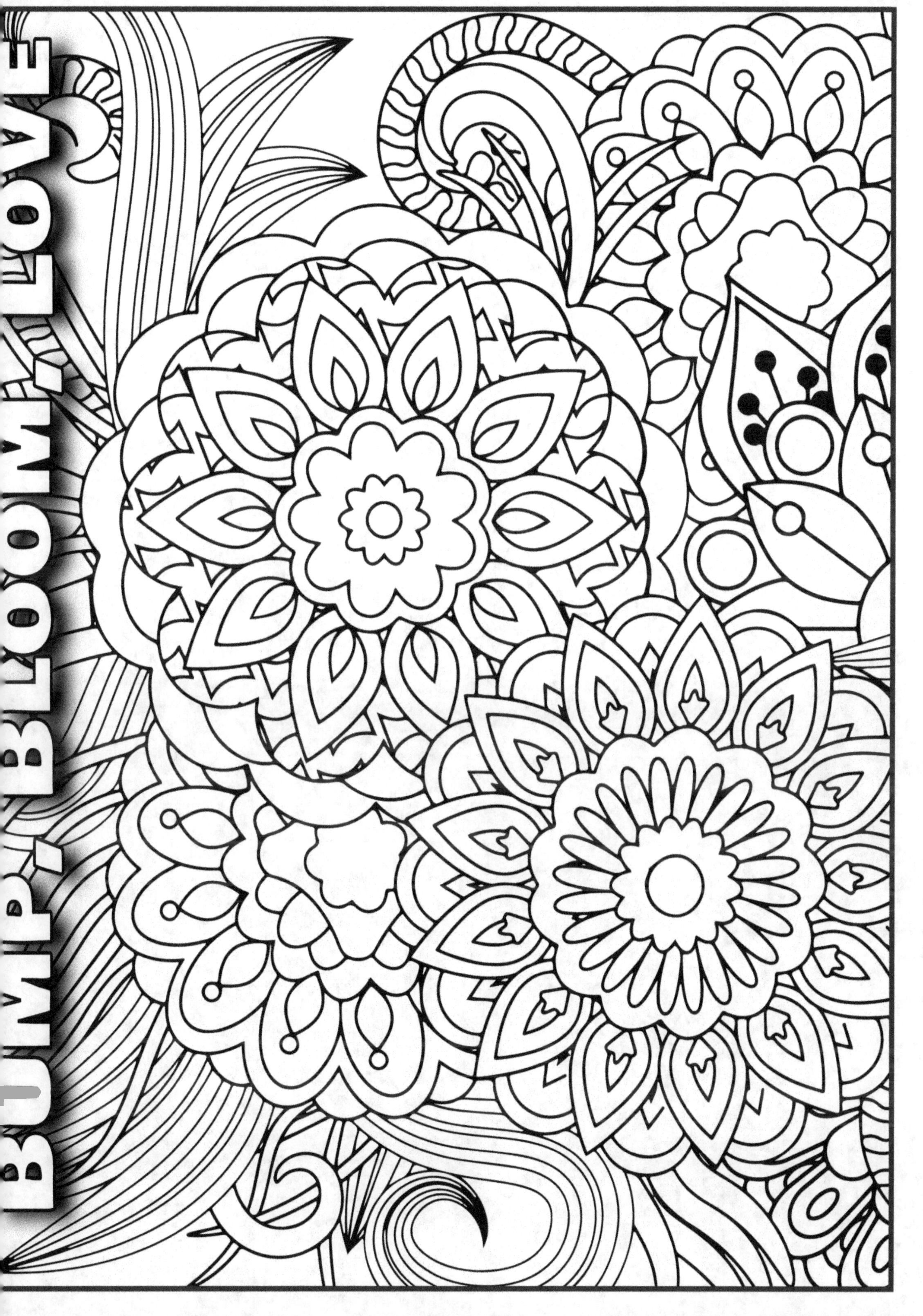
BUMP, BLOOM, LOVE

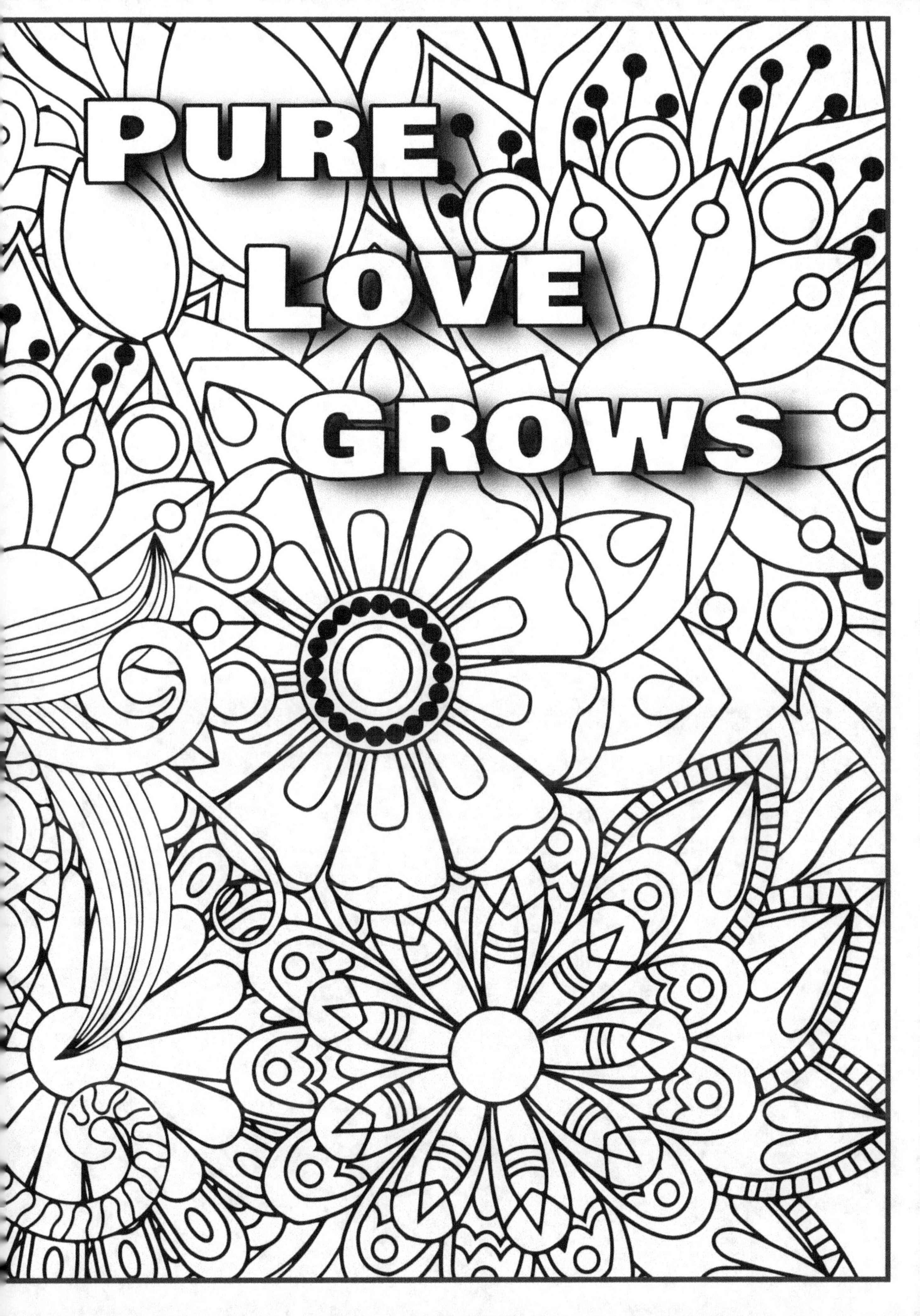

PURE
LOVE
GROWS

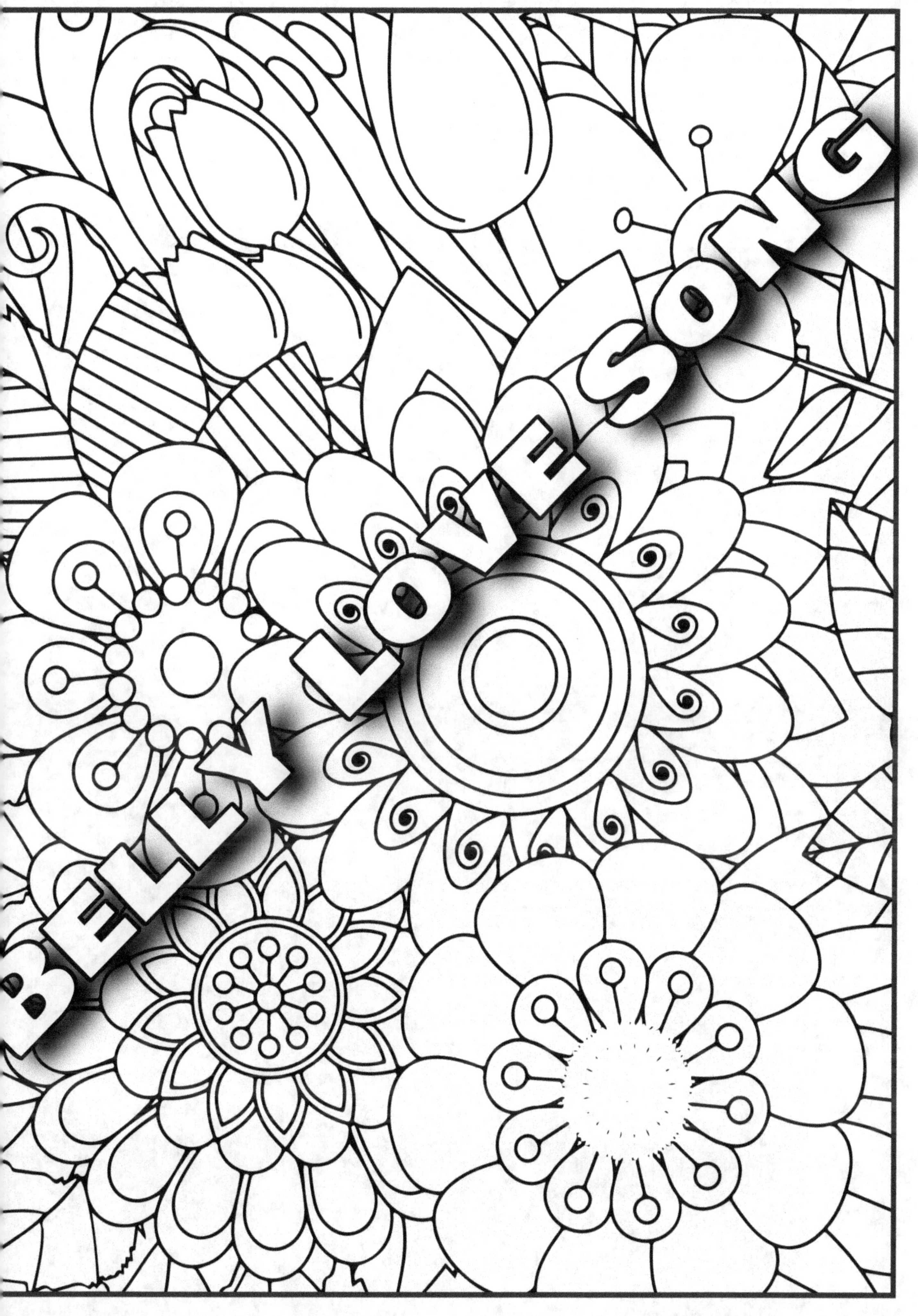

BELLY LOVE SONG

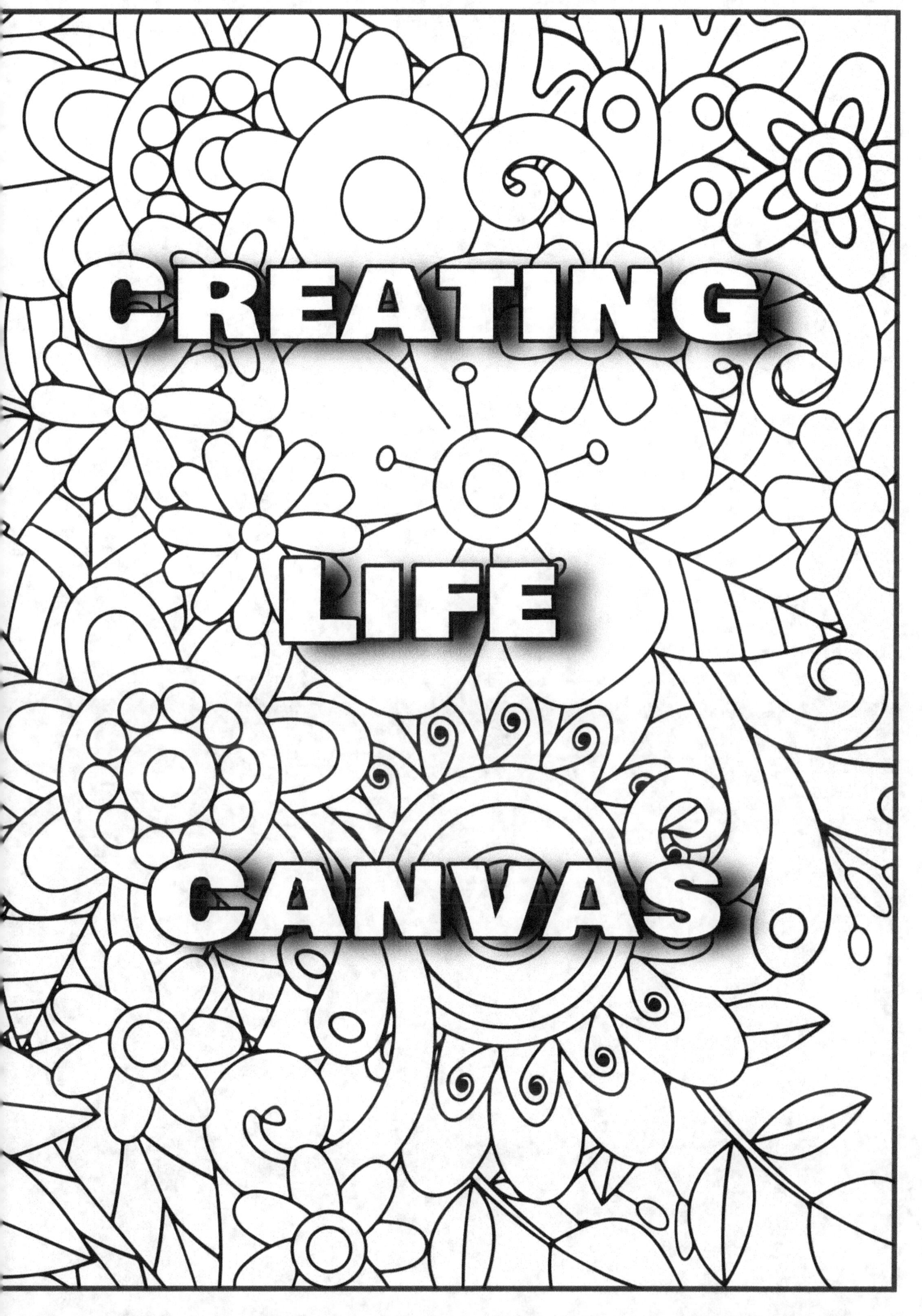

CREATING
LIFE
CANVAS

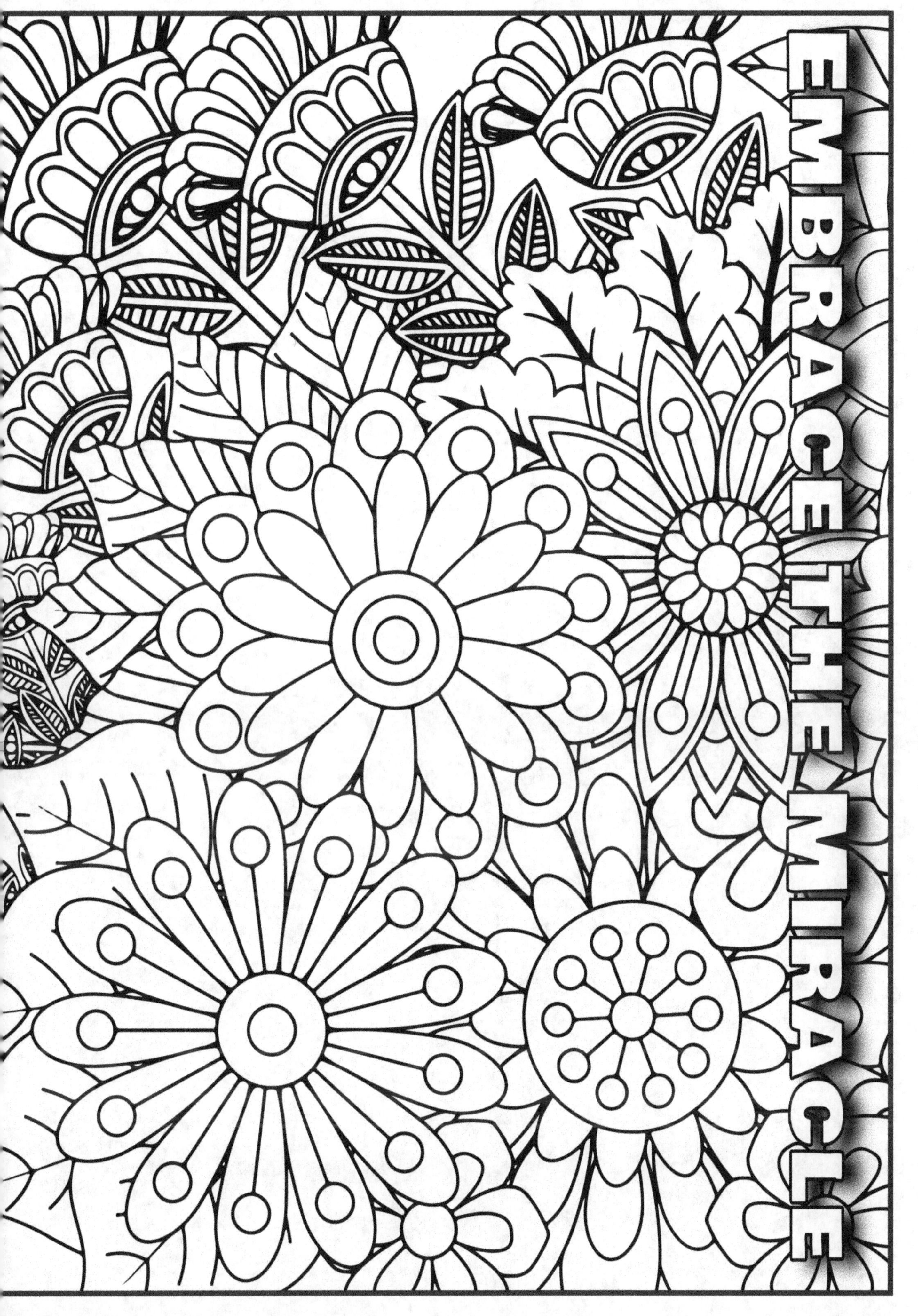
EMBRACE THE MIRACLE

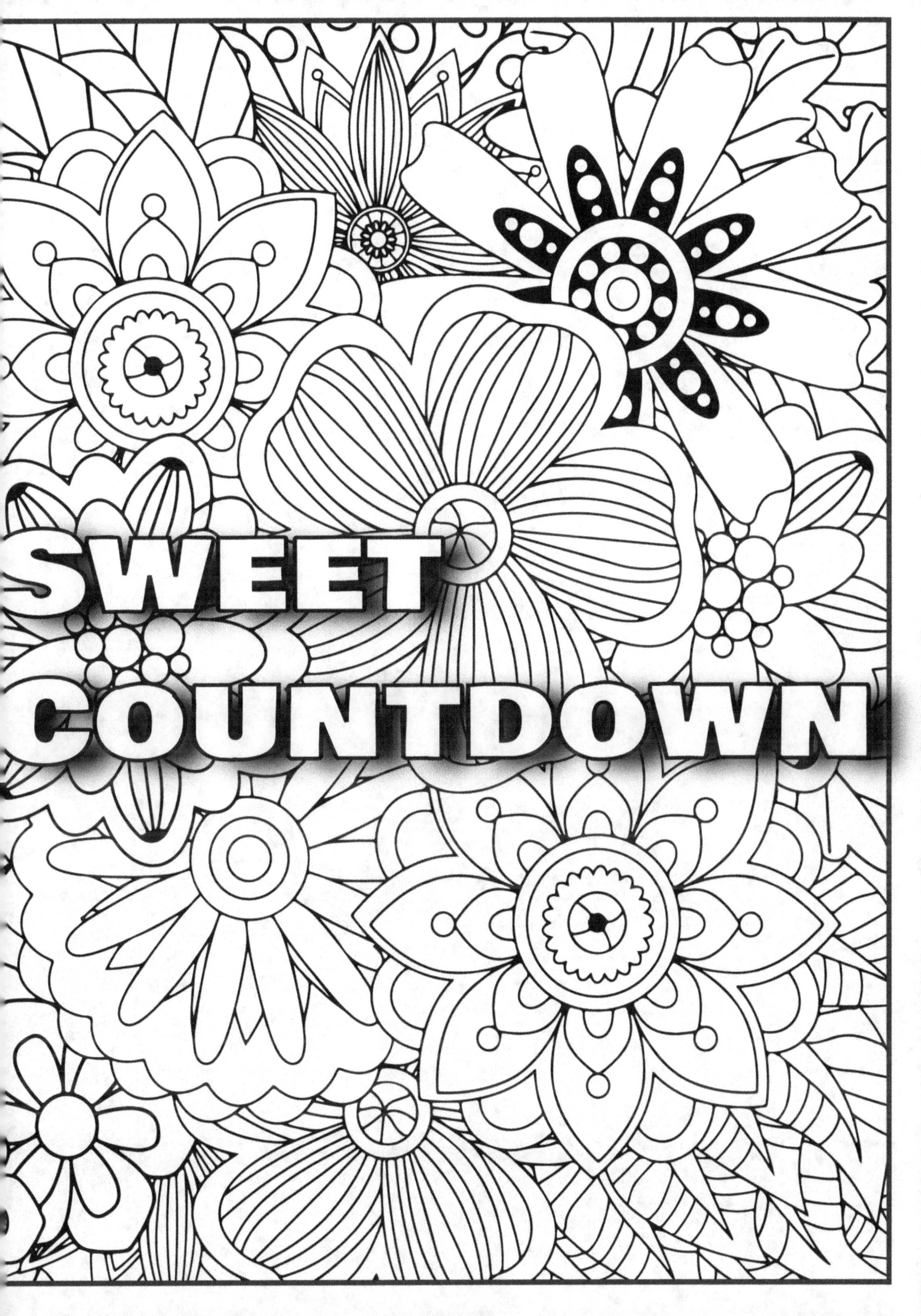
SWEET
COUNTDOWN

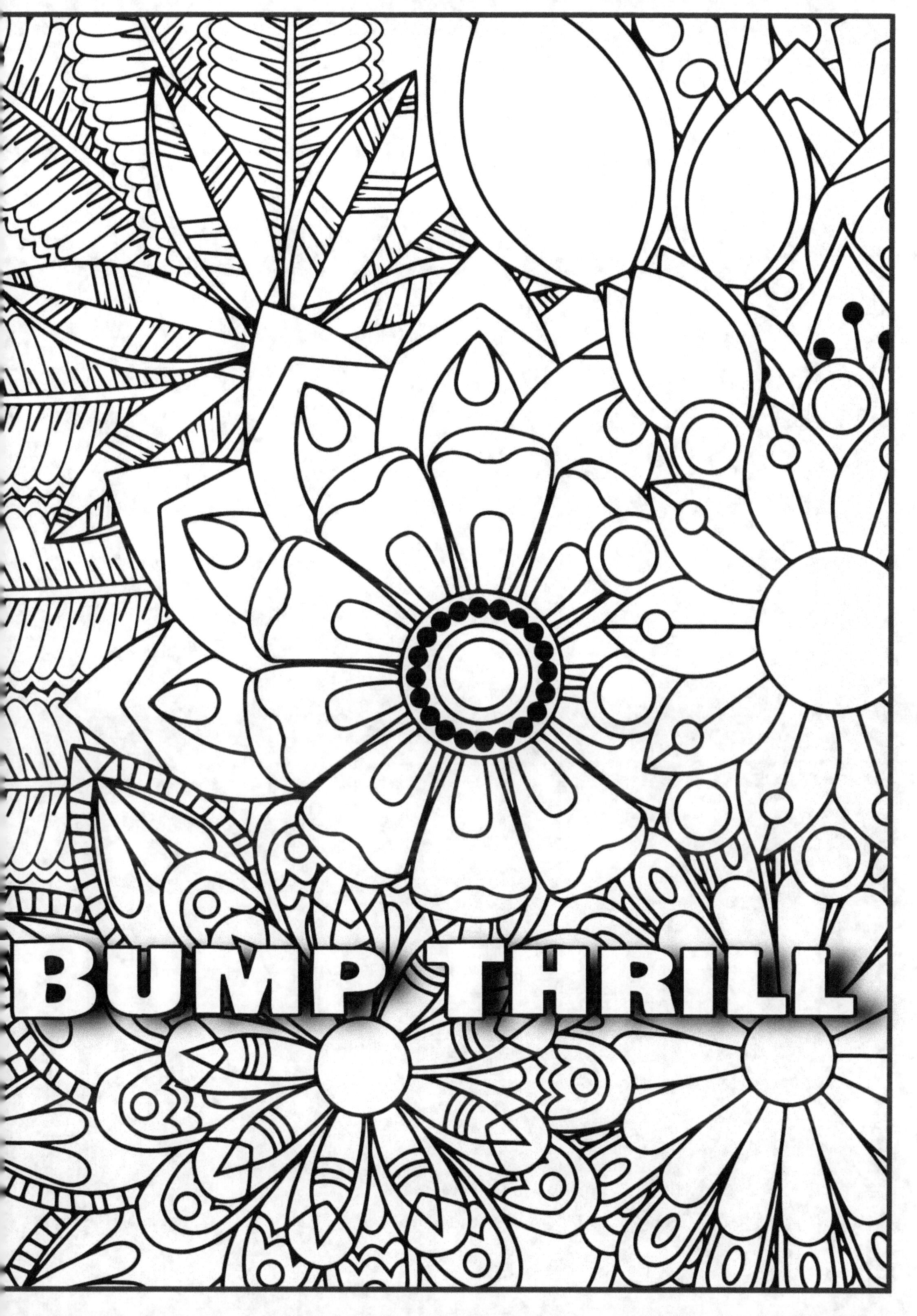
BUMP THRILL

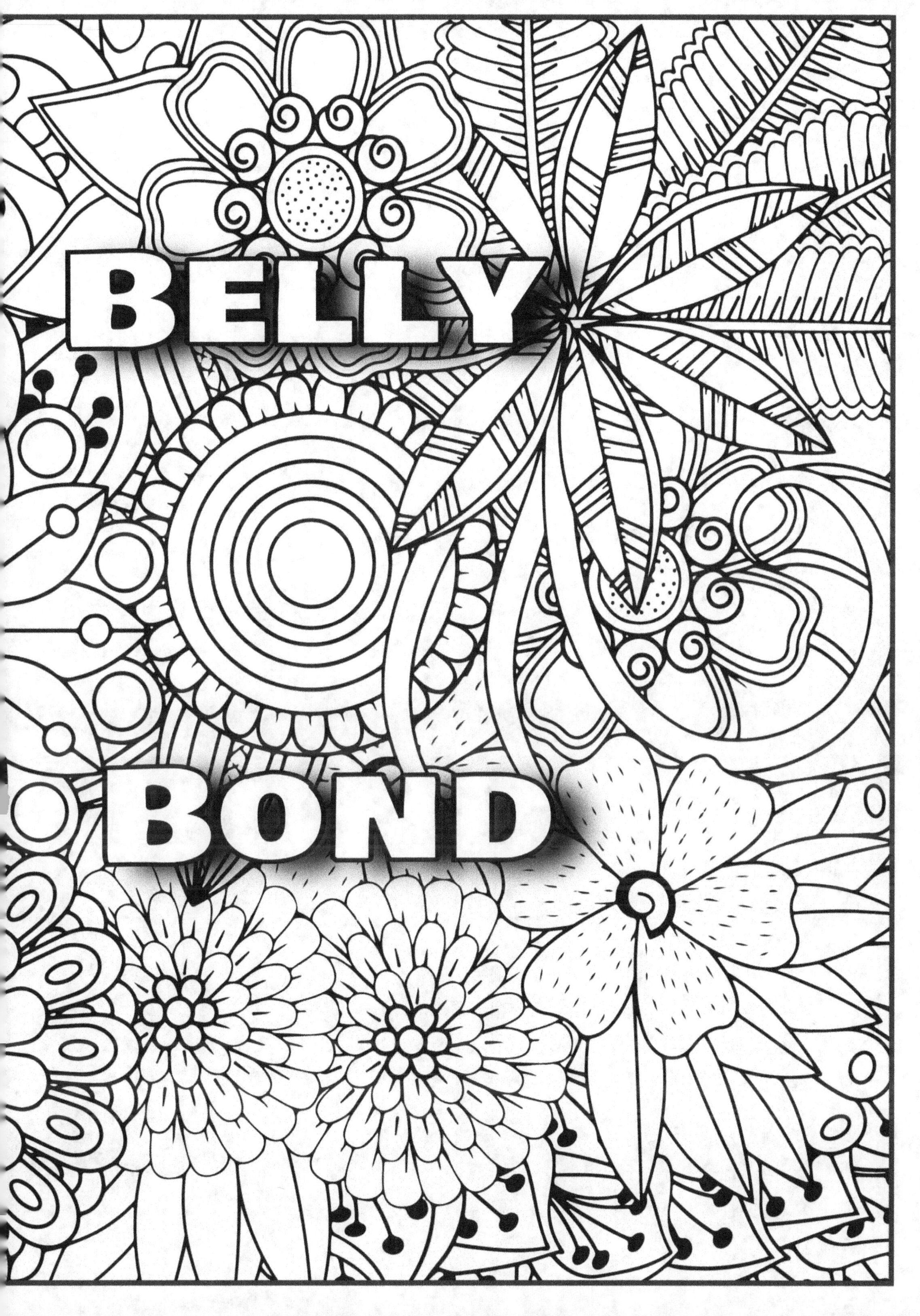
BELLY
BOND

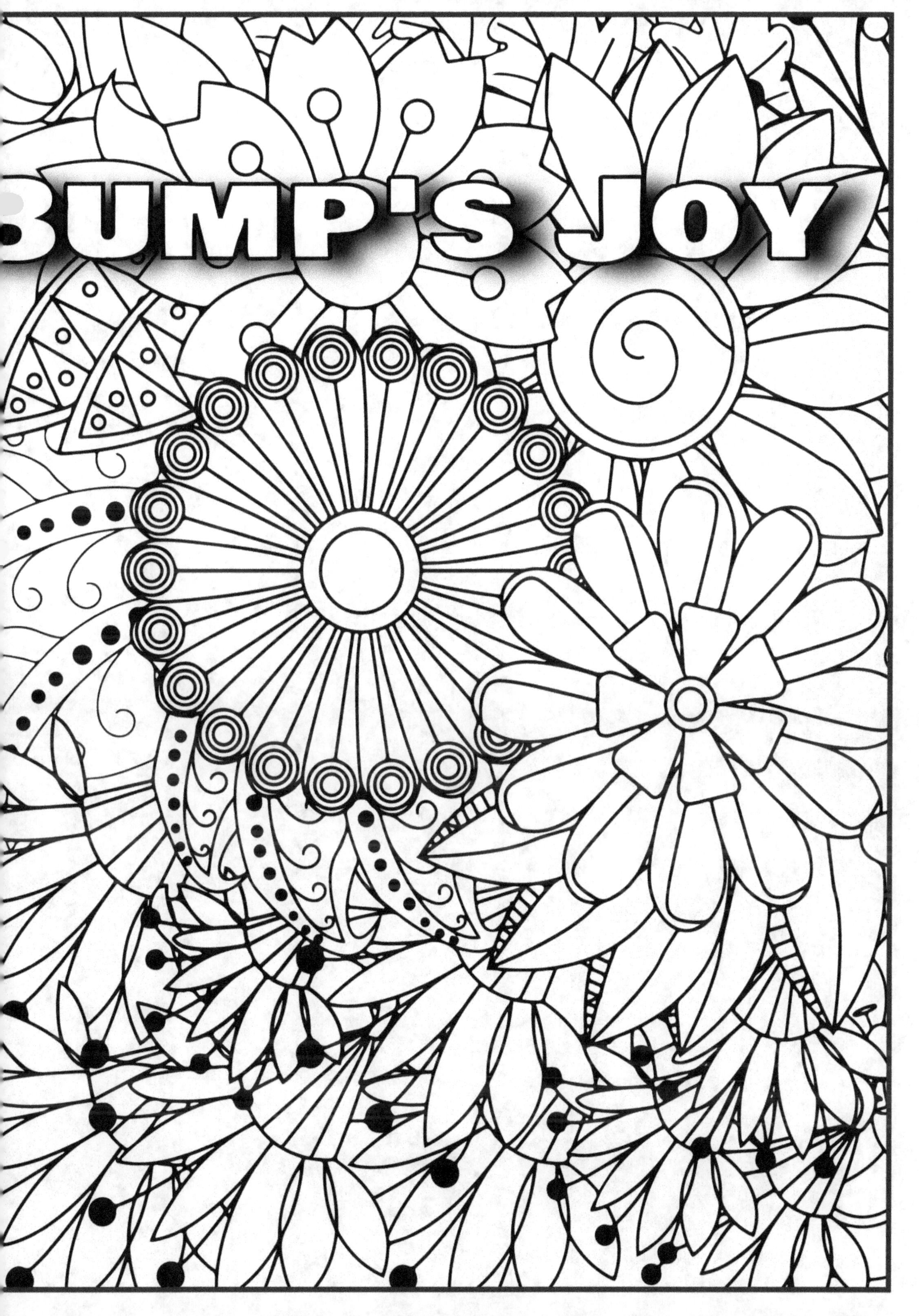
BUMP'S JOY

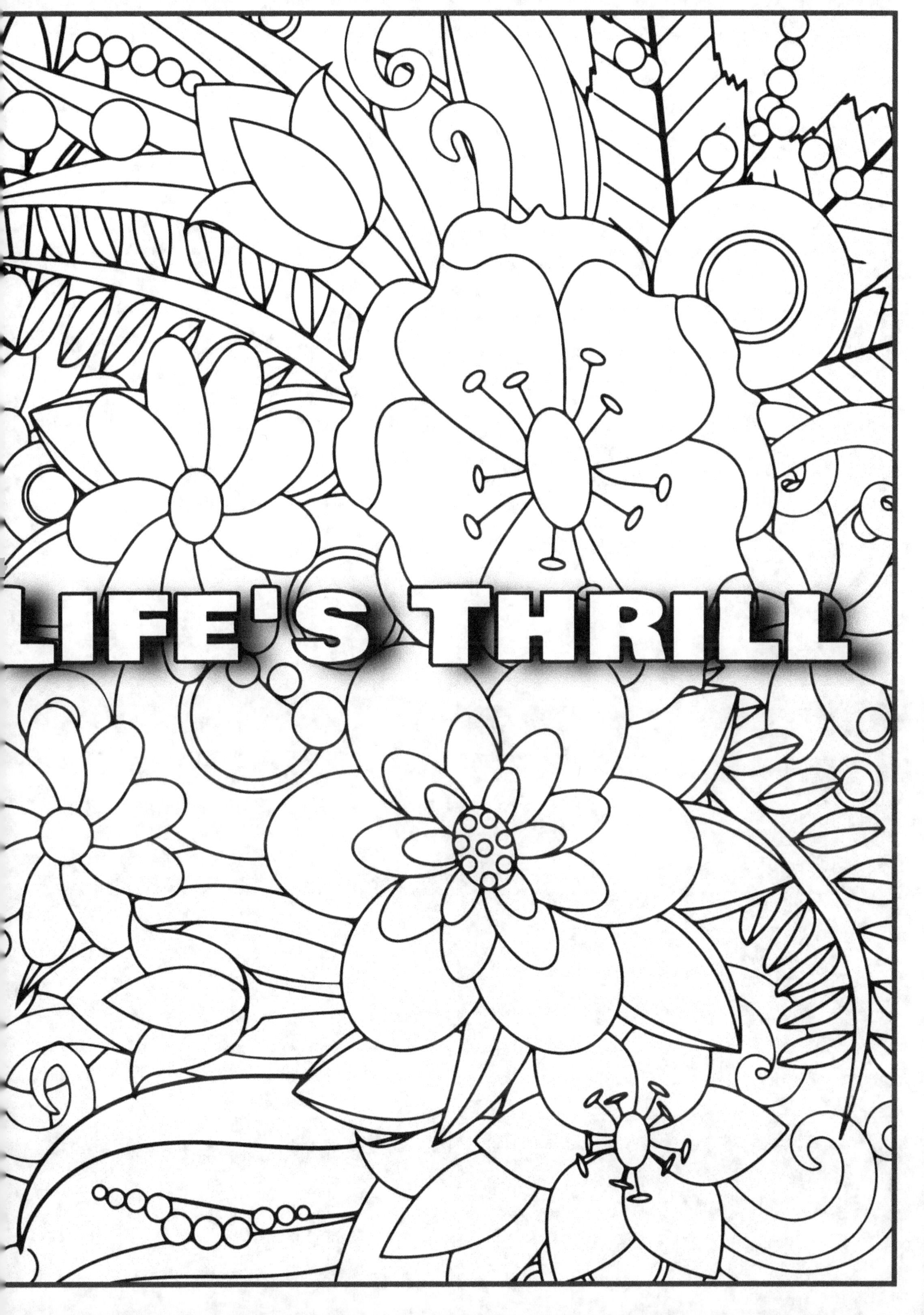
LIFE'S THRILL

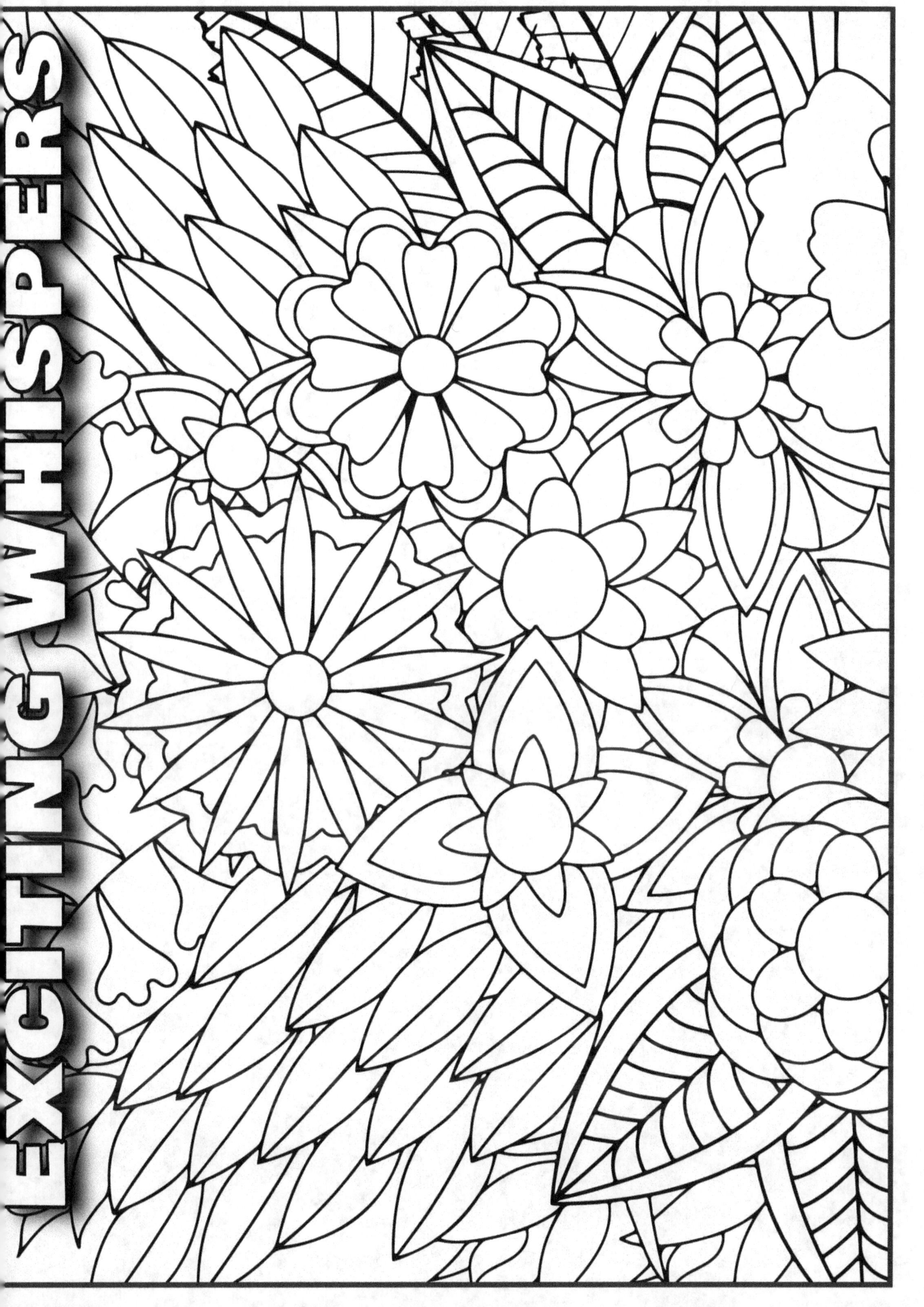
EXCITING WHISPERS

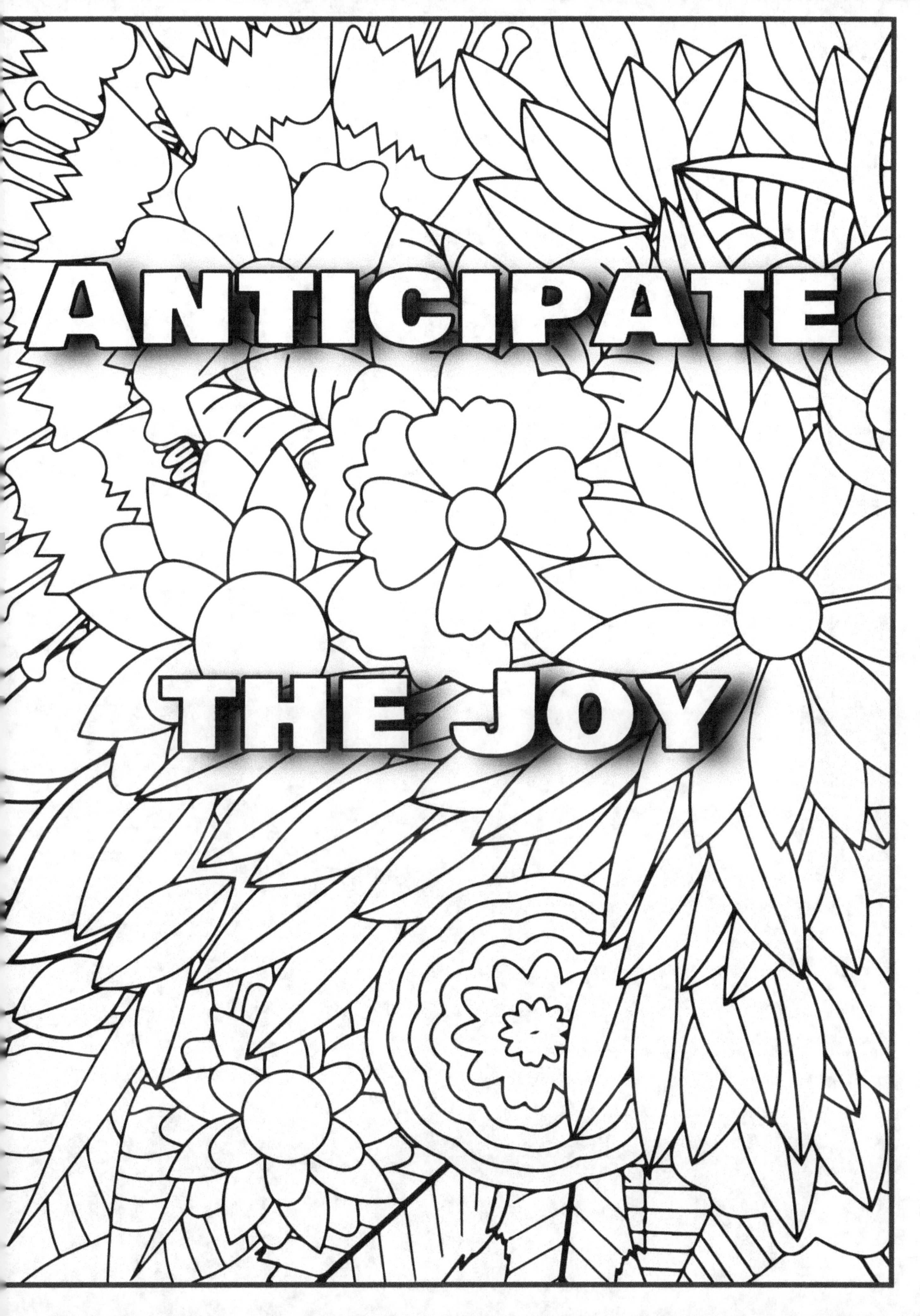

ANTICIPATE
THE JOY

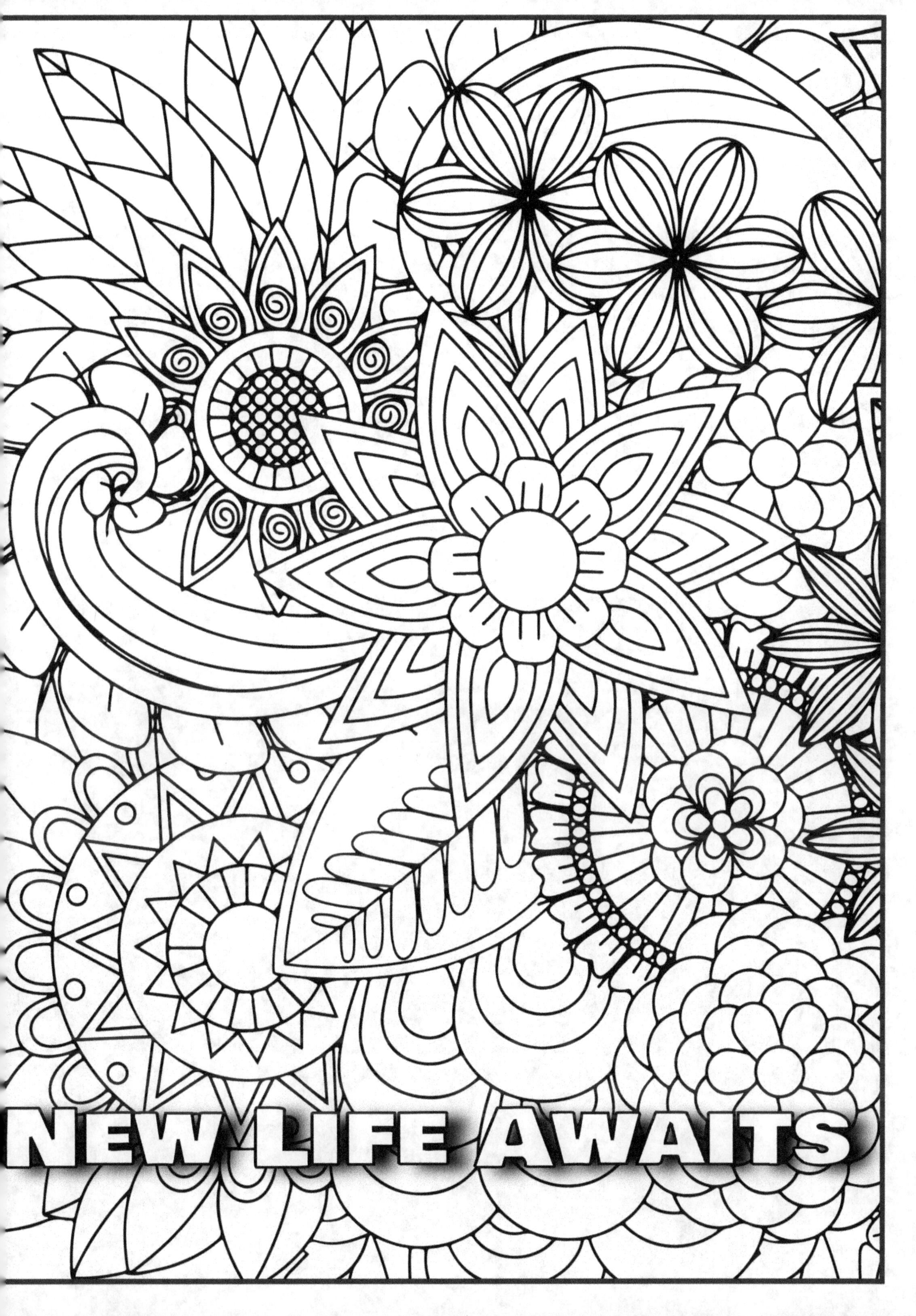
NEW LIFE AWAITS

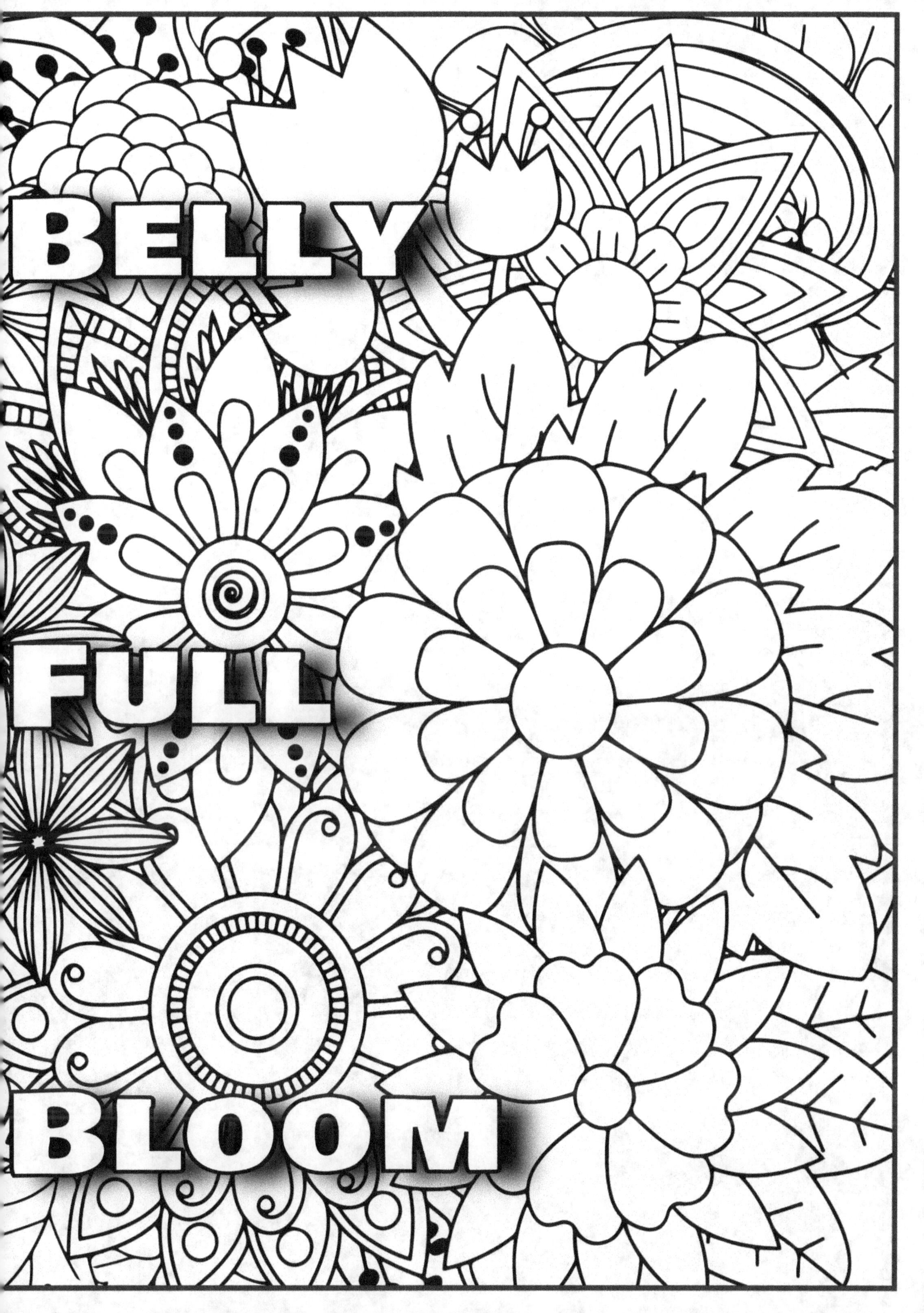
BELLY
FULL
BLOOM

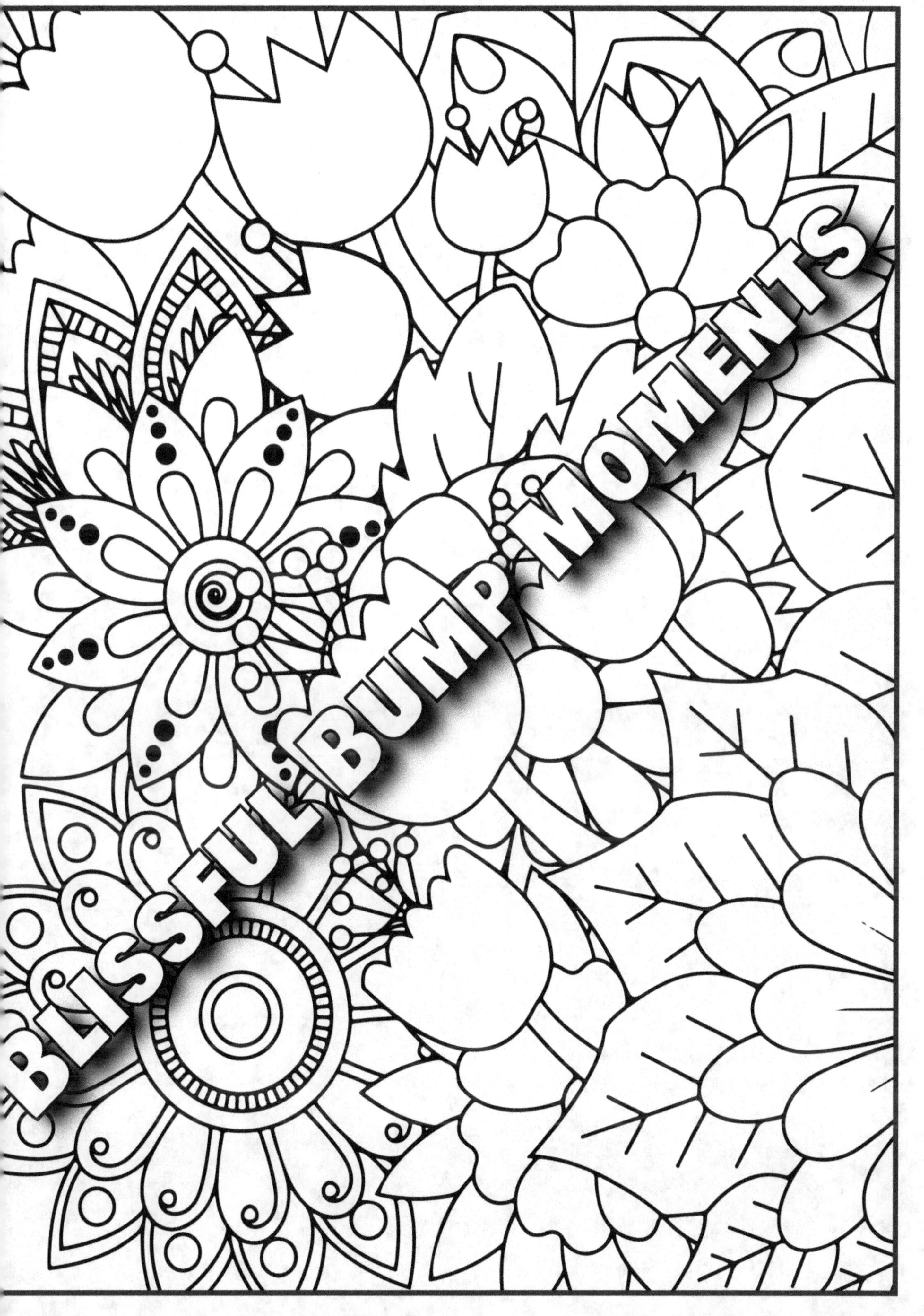
BLISSFUL BUMP MOMENTS

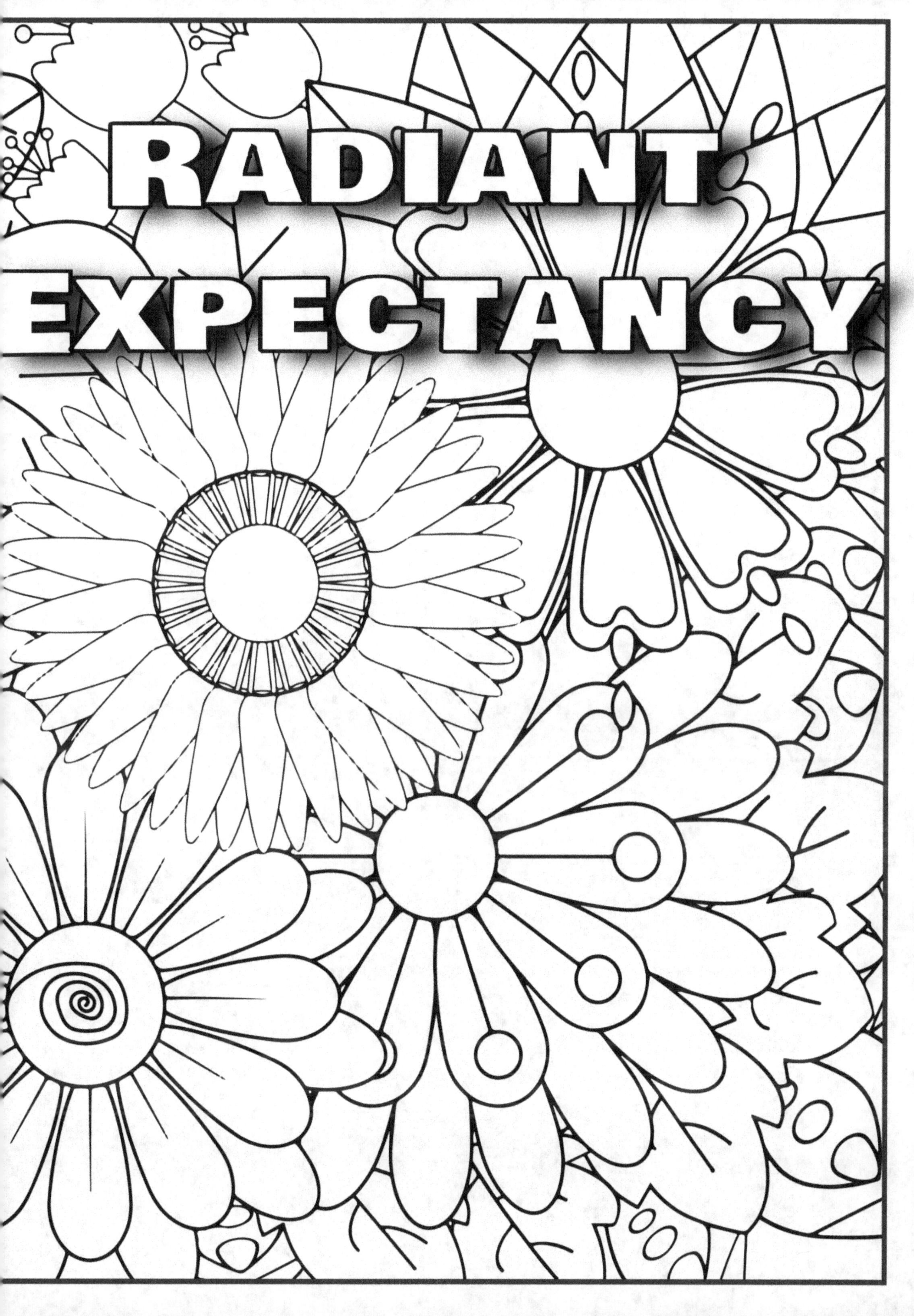

RADIANT
EXPECTANCY

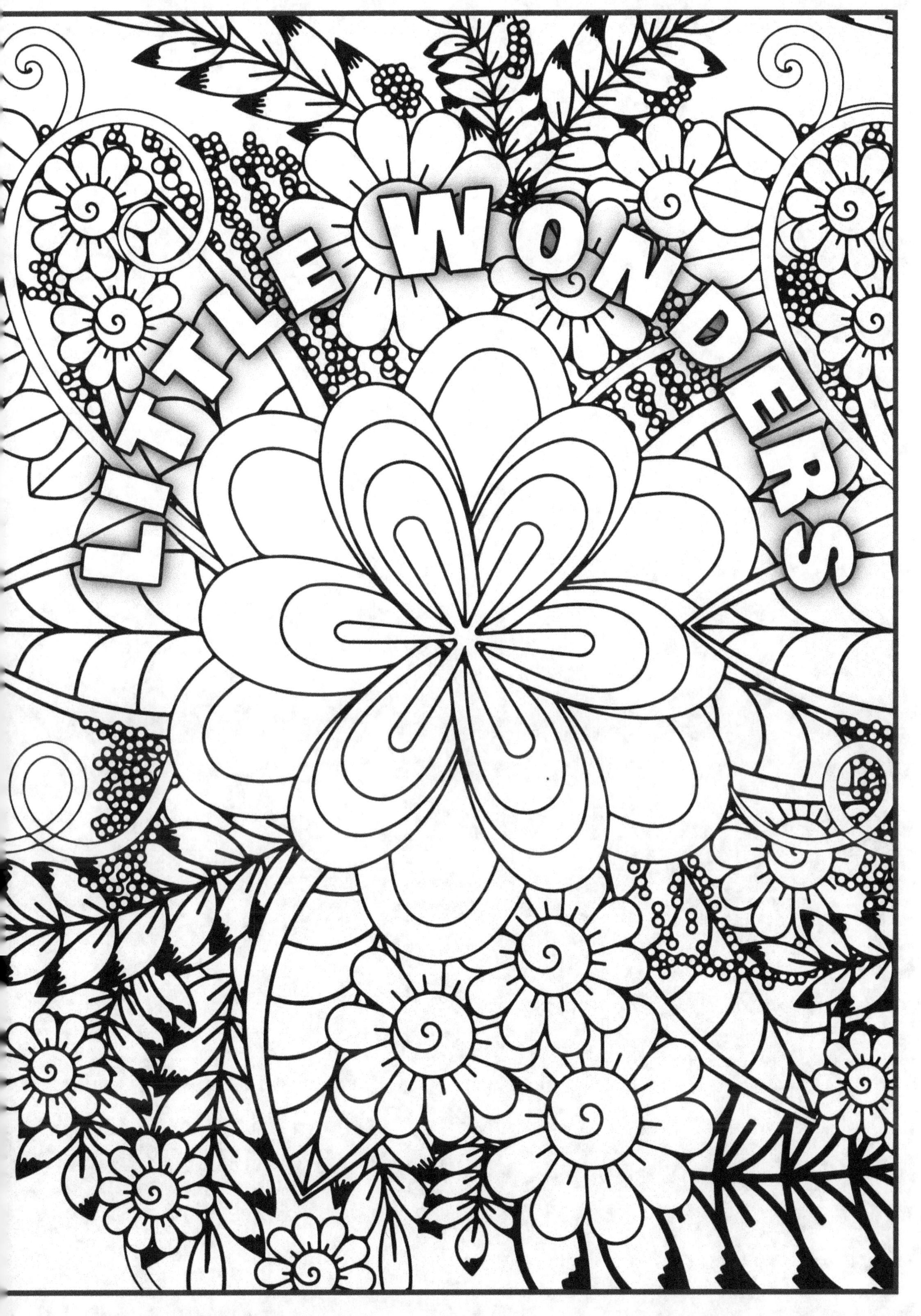

LITTLE WONDERS

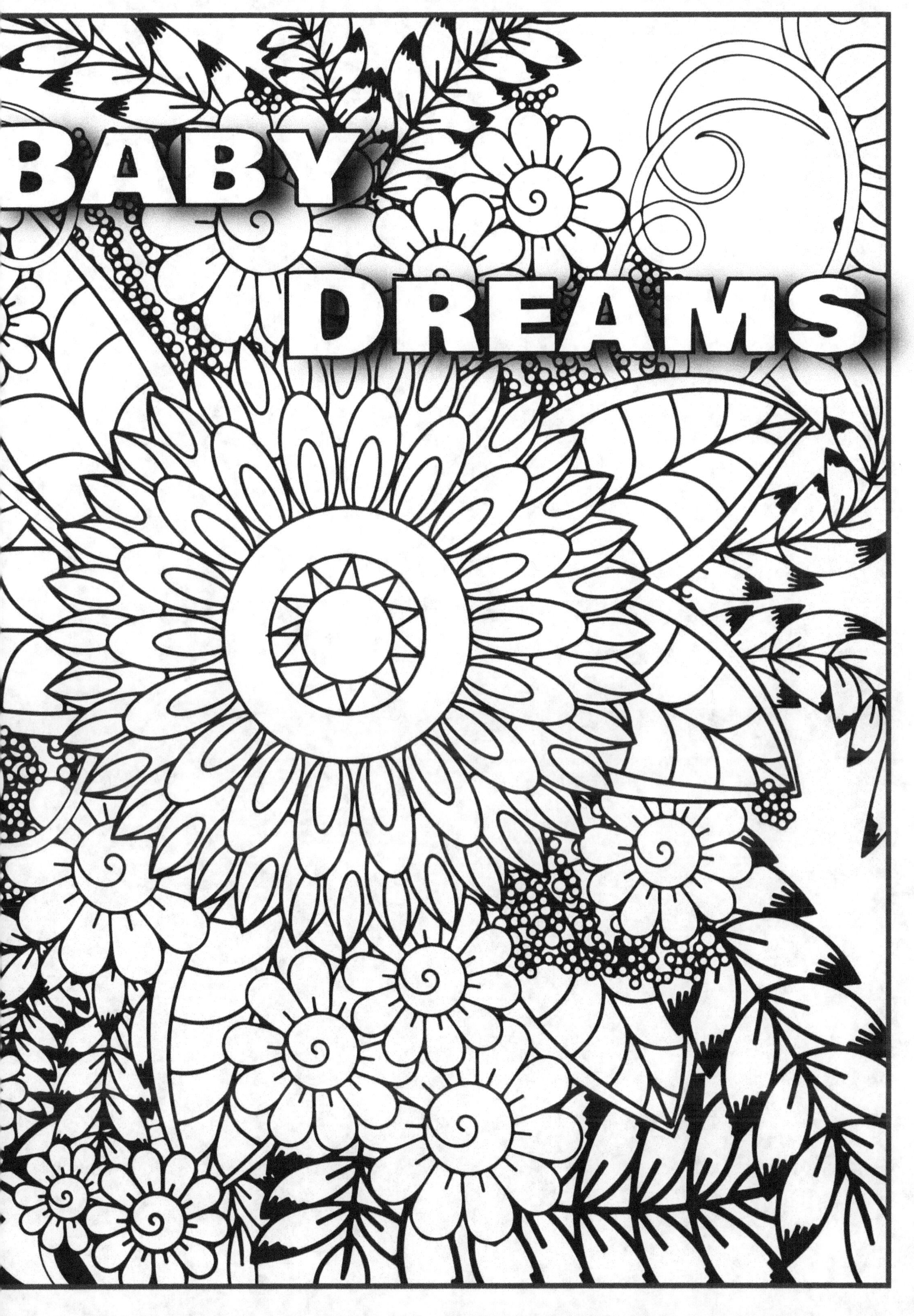
BABY
DREAMS

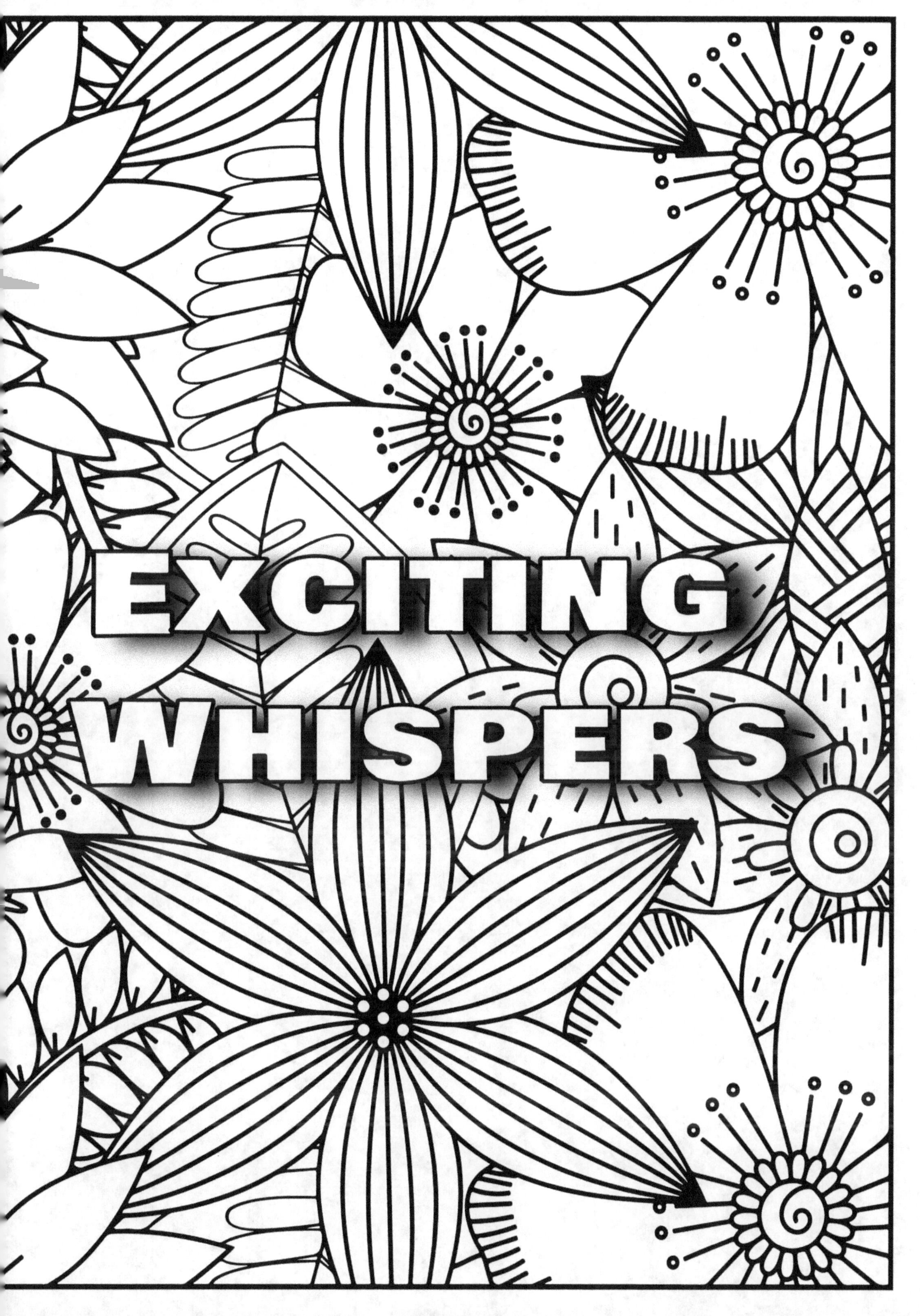

EXCITING
WHISPERS

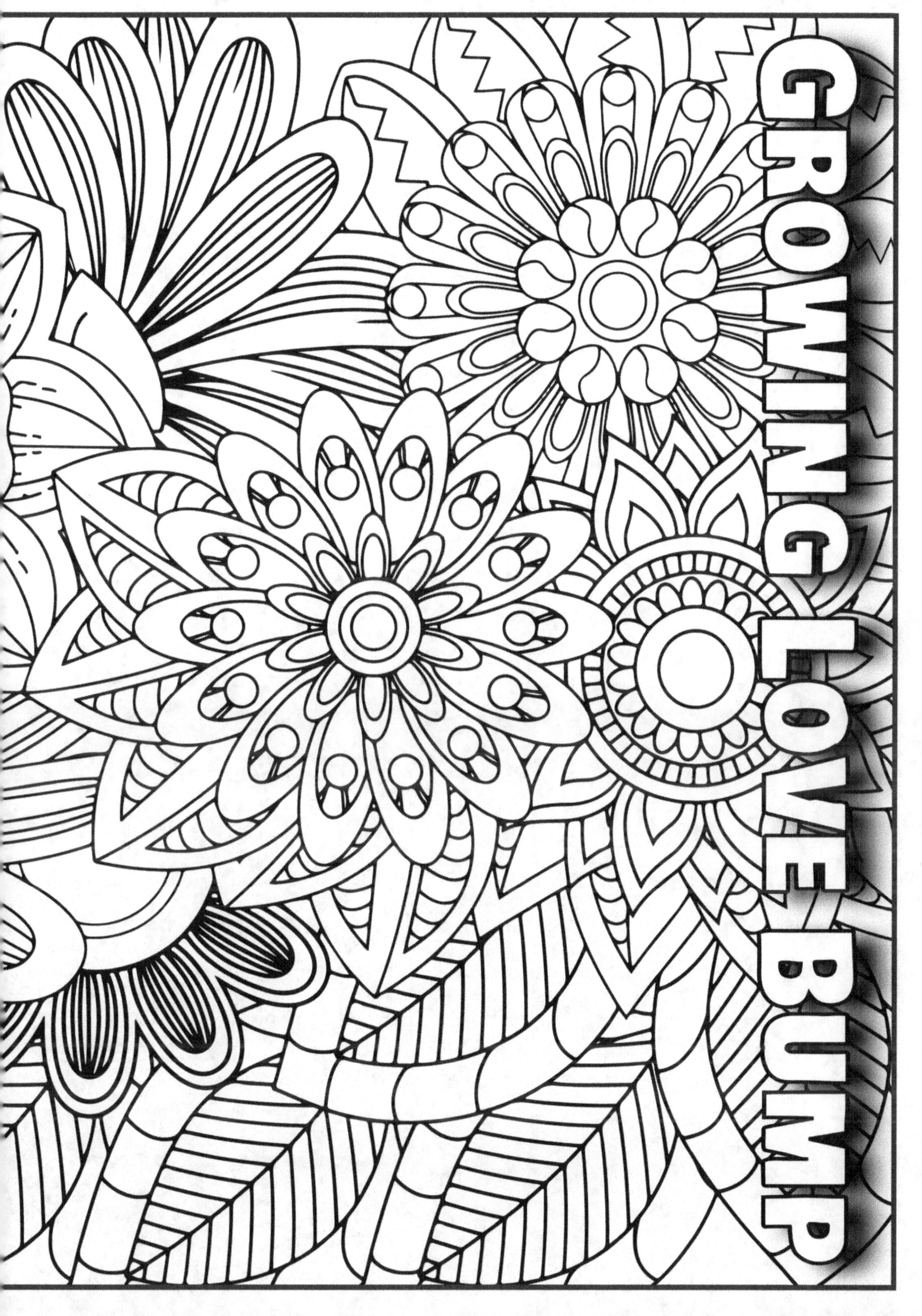

GROWING LOVE BUMP

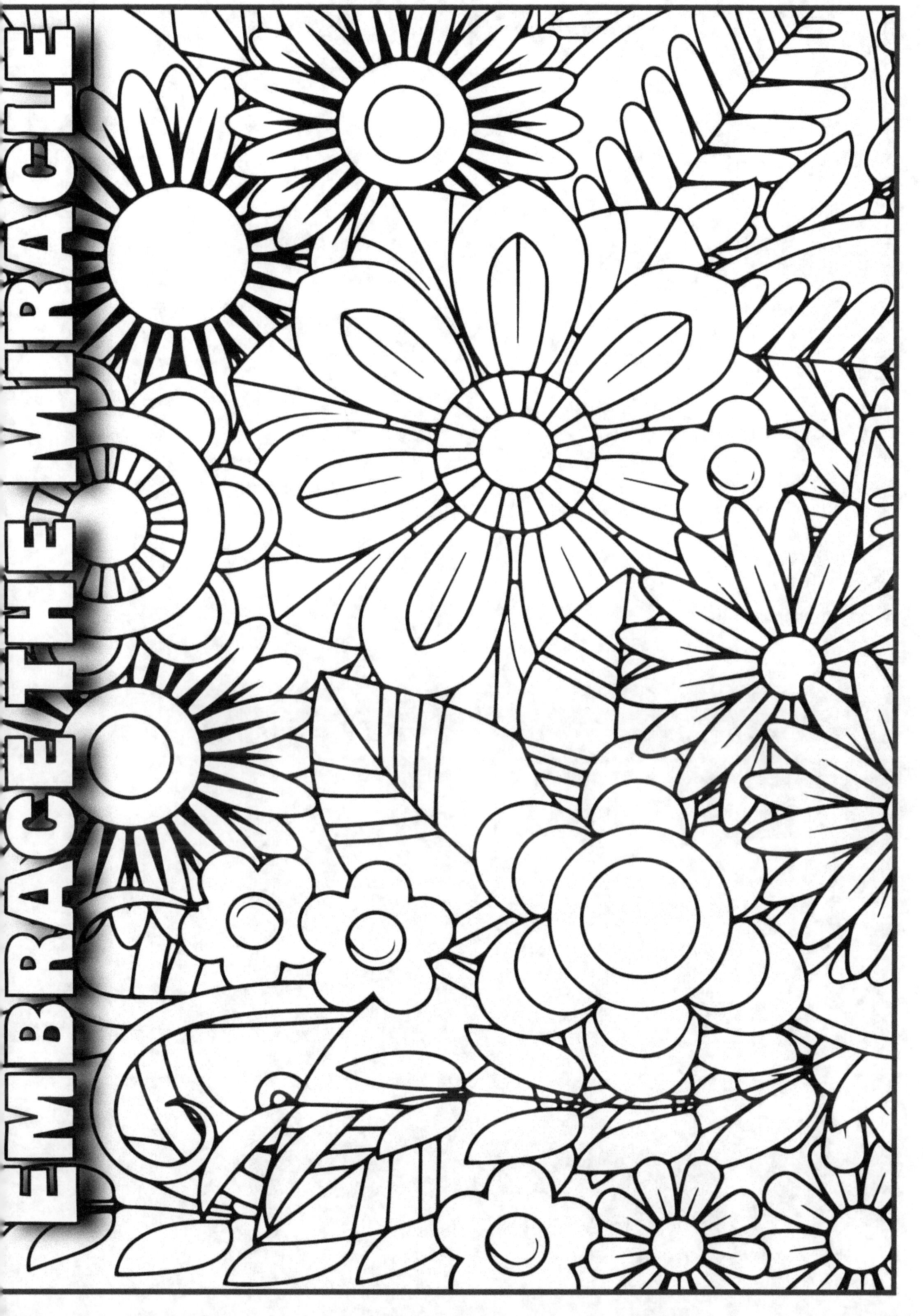

EMBRACE THE MIRACLE

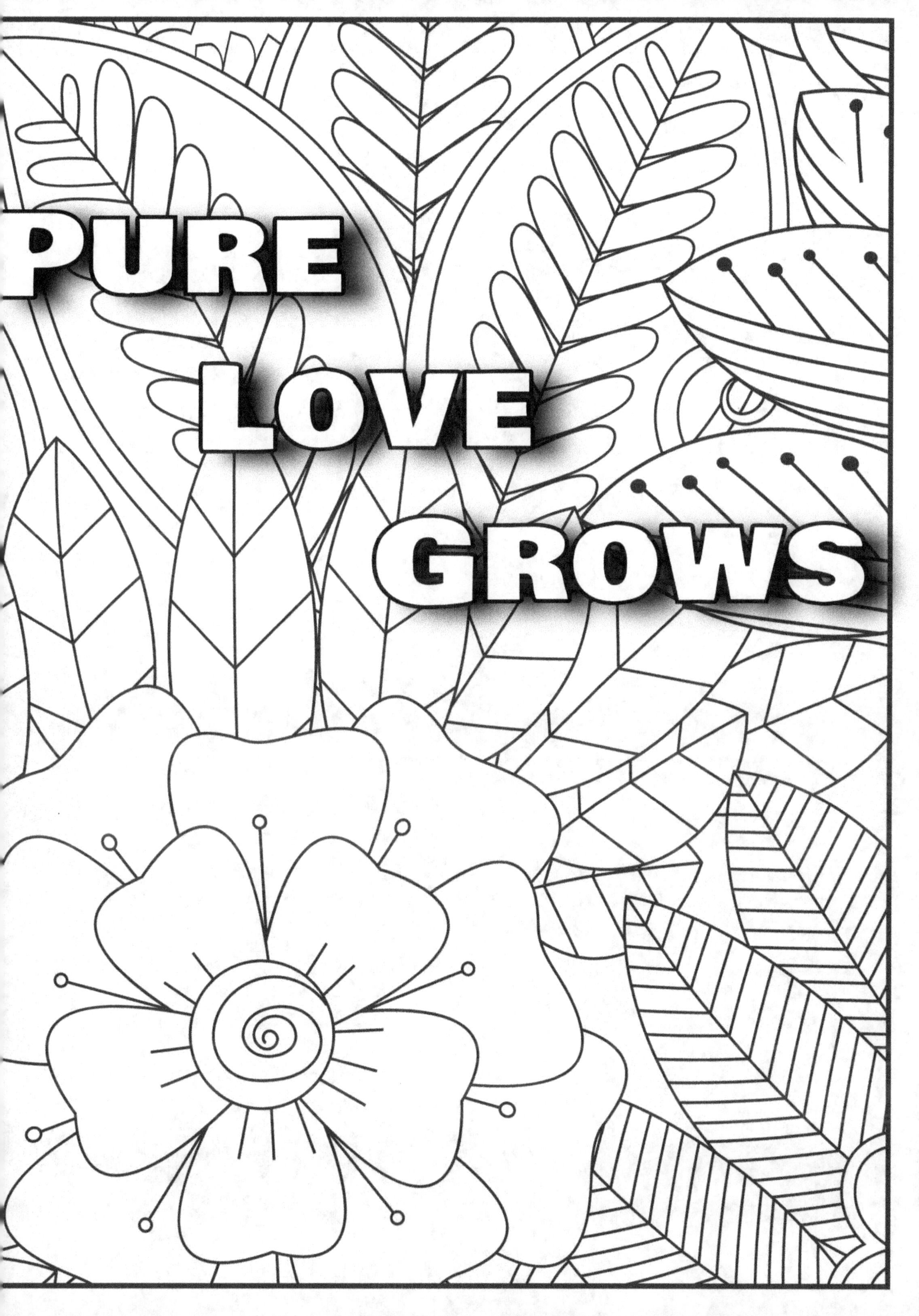

PURE
LOVE
GROWS

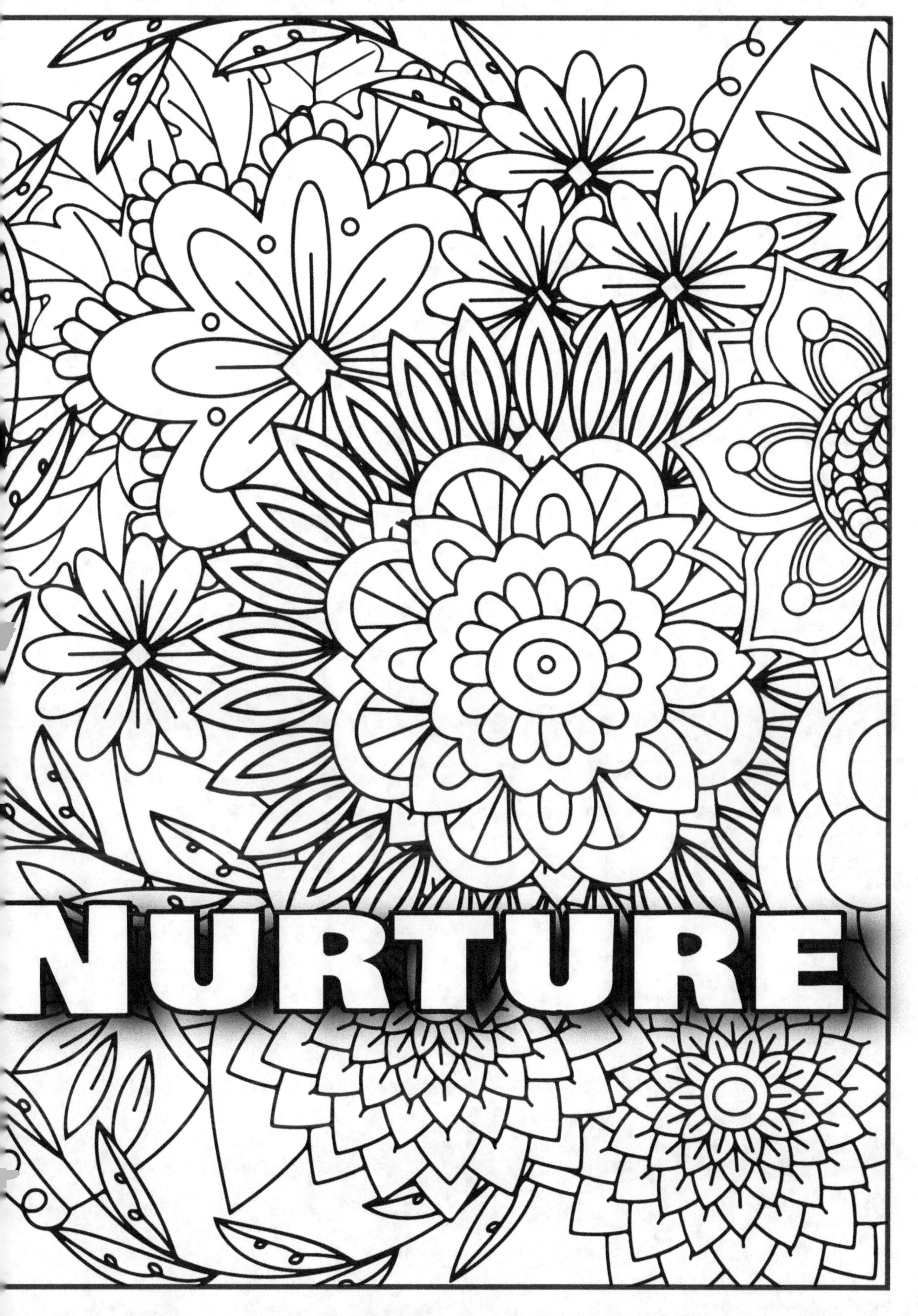
NURTURE

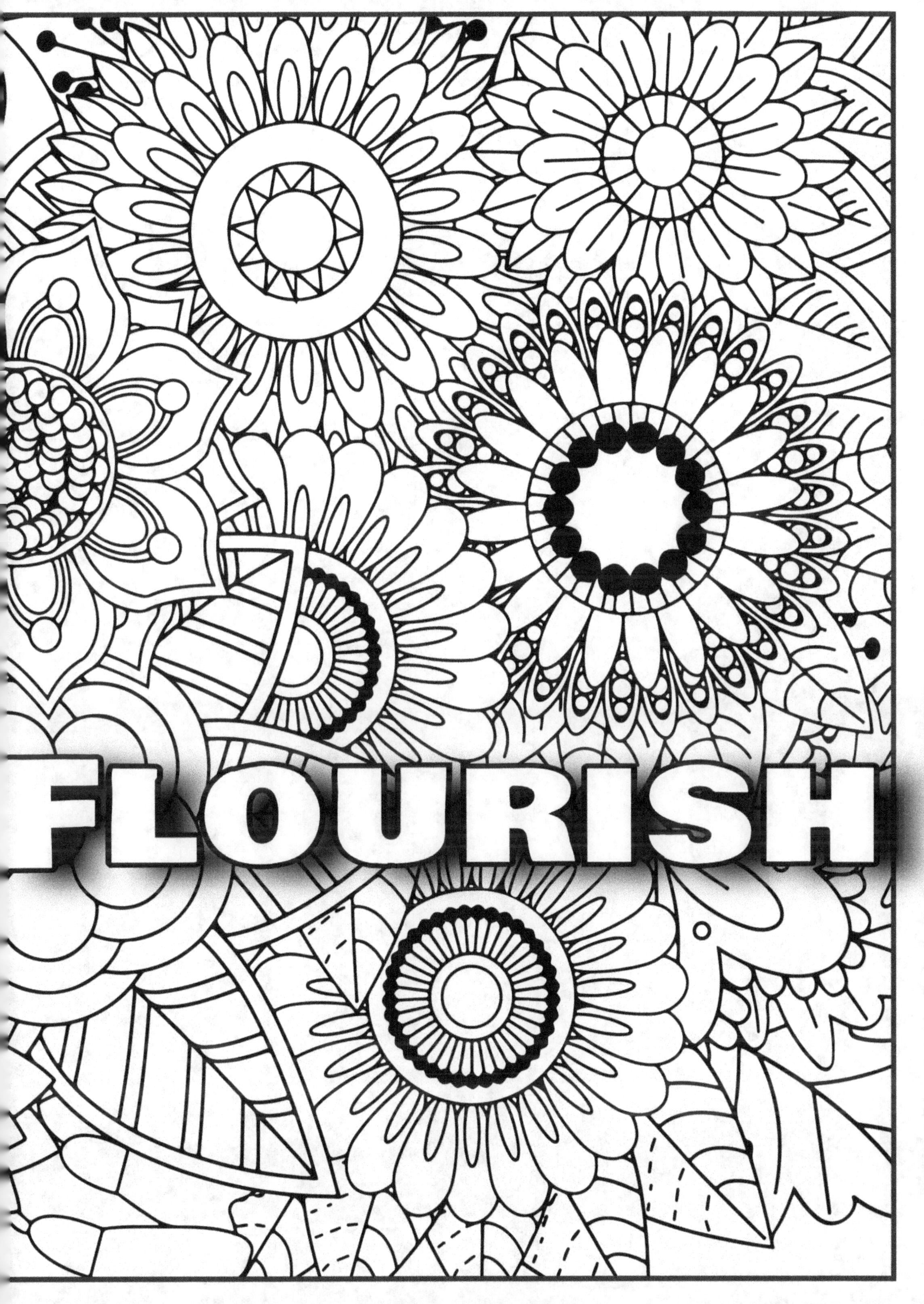
FLOURISH

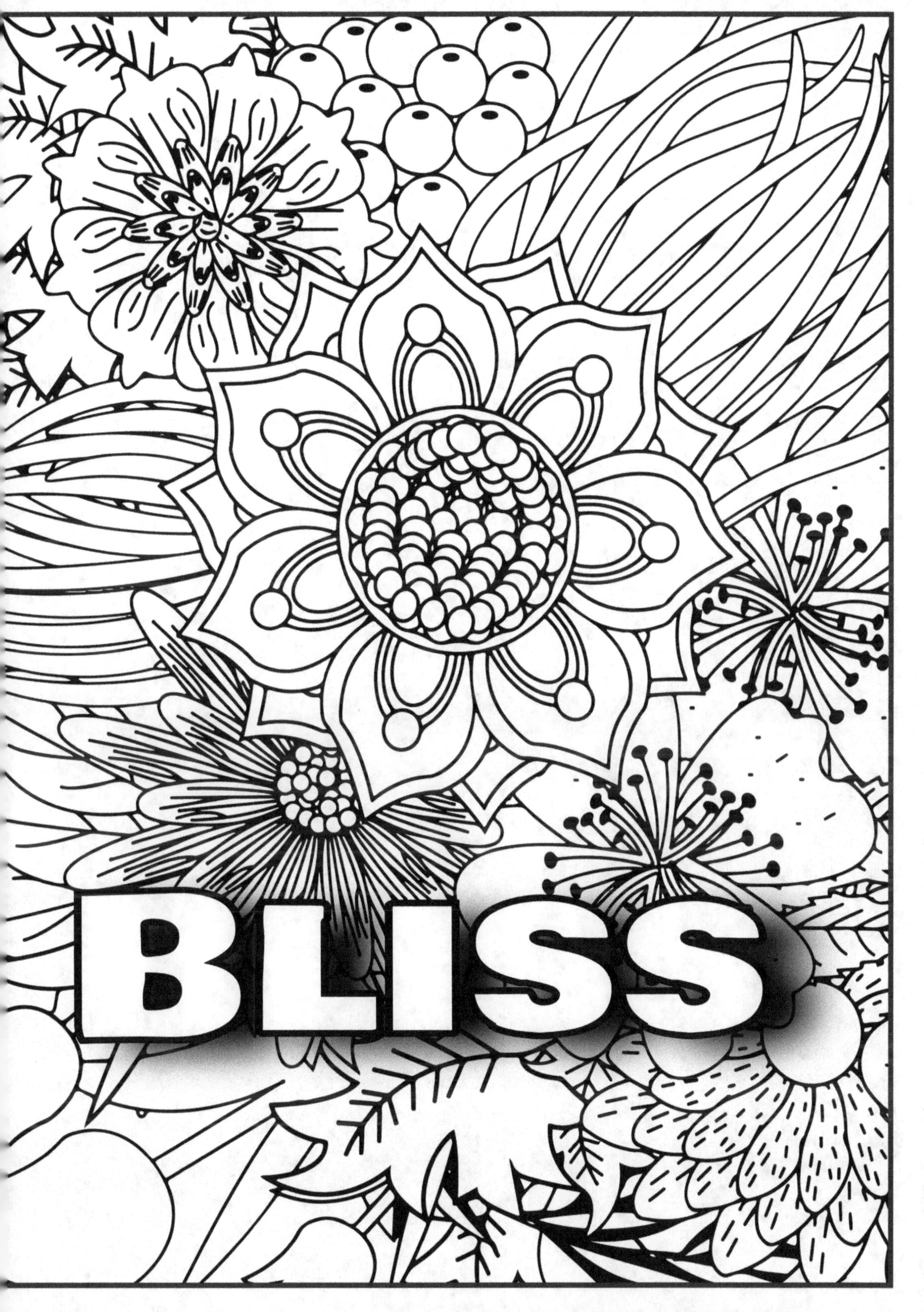
BLISS

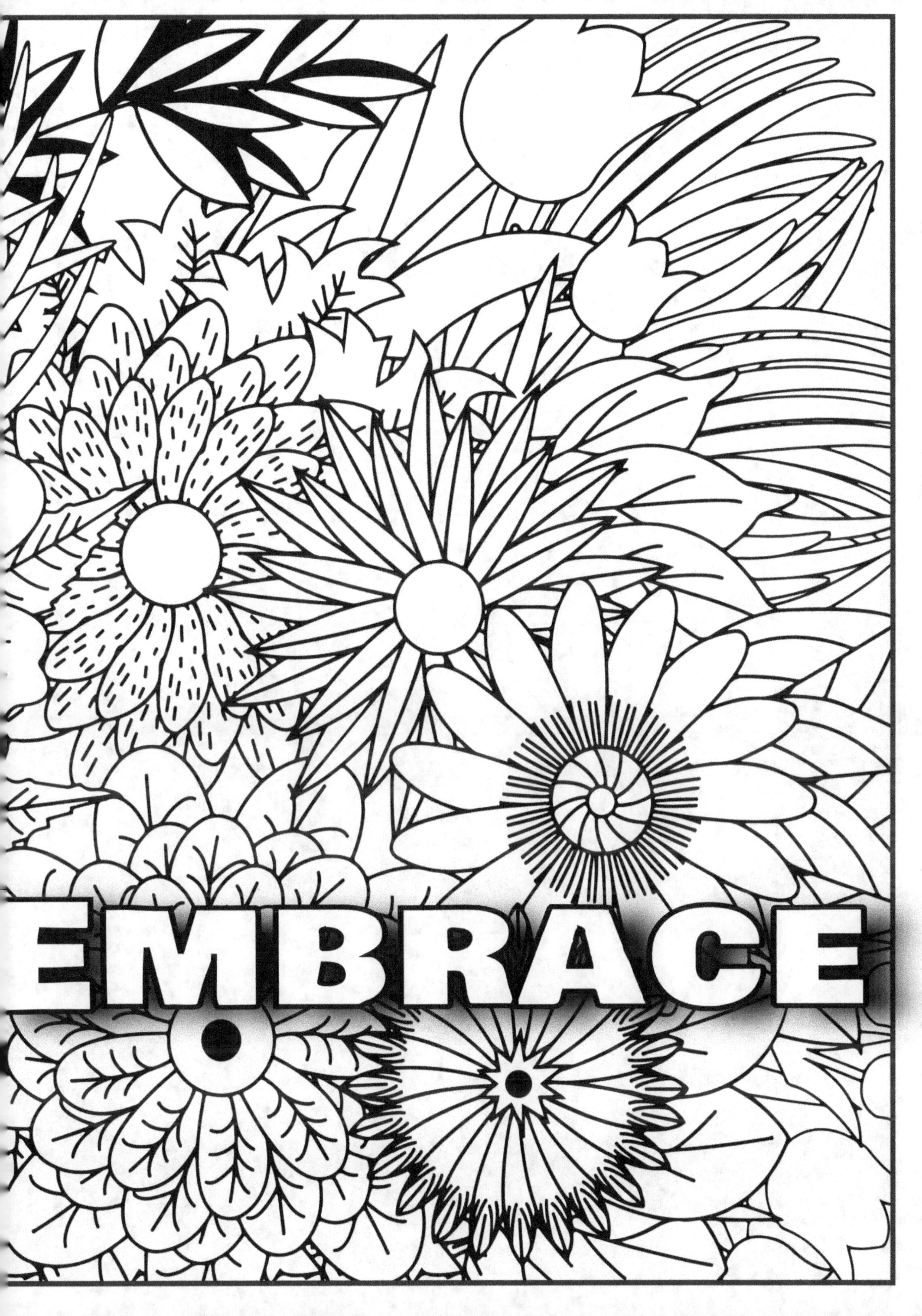
EMBRACE

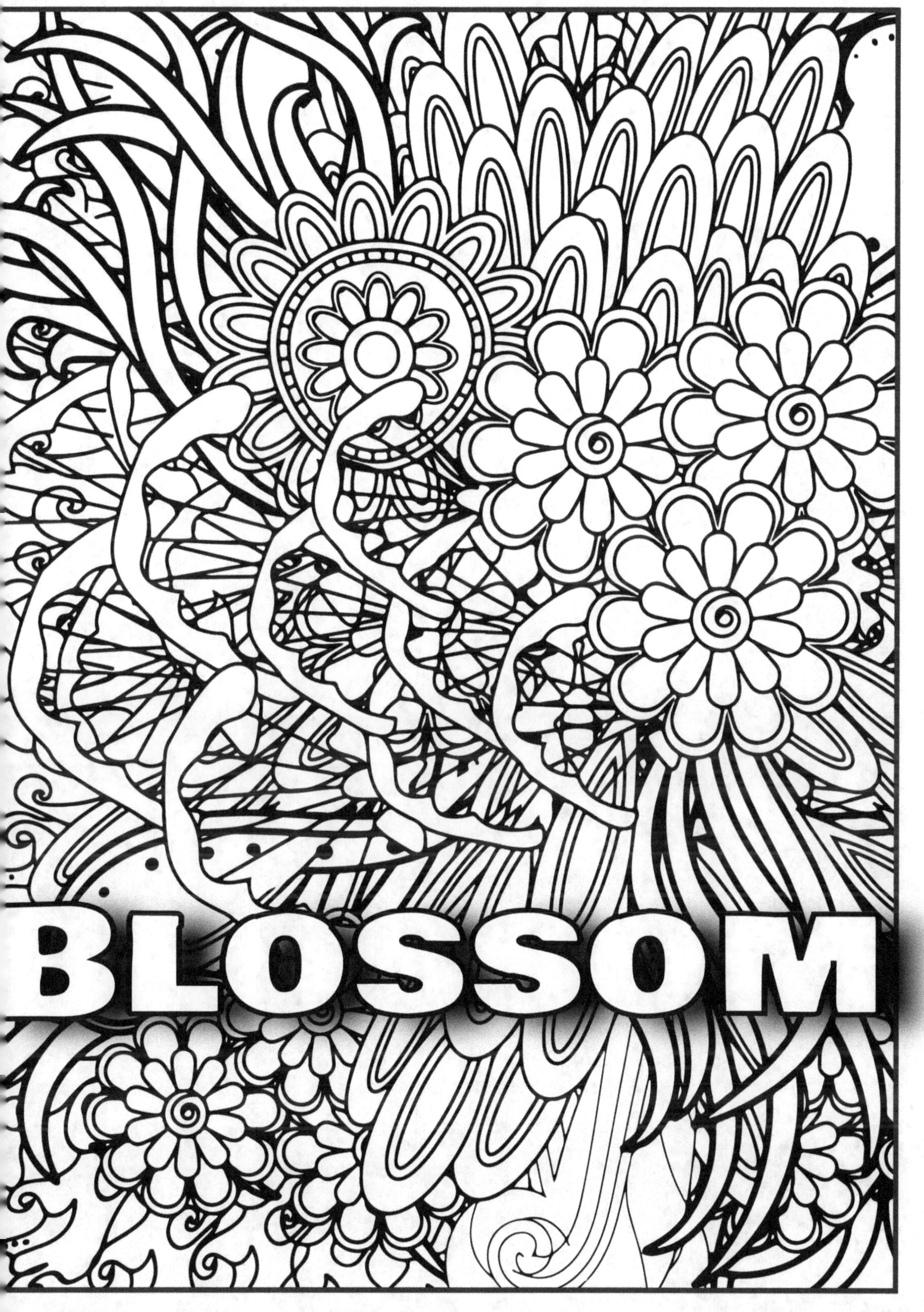
BLOSSOM

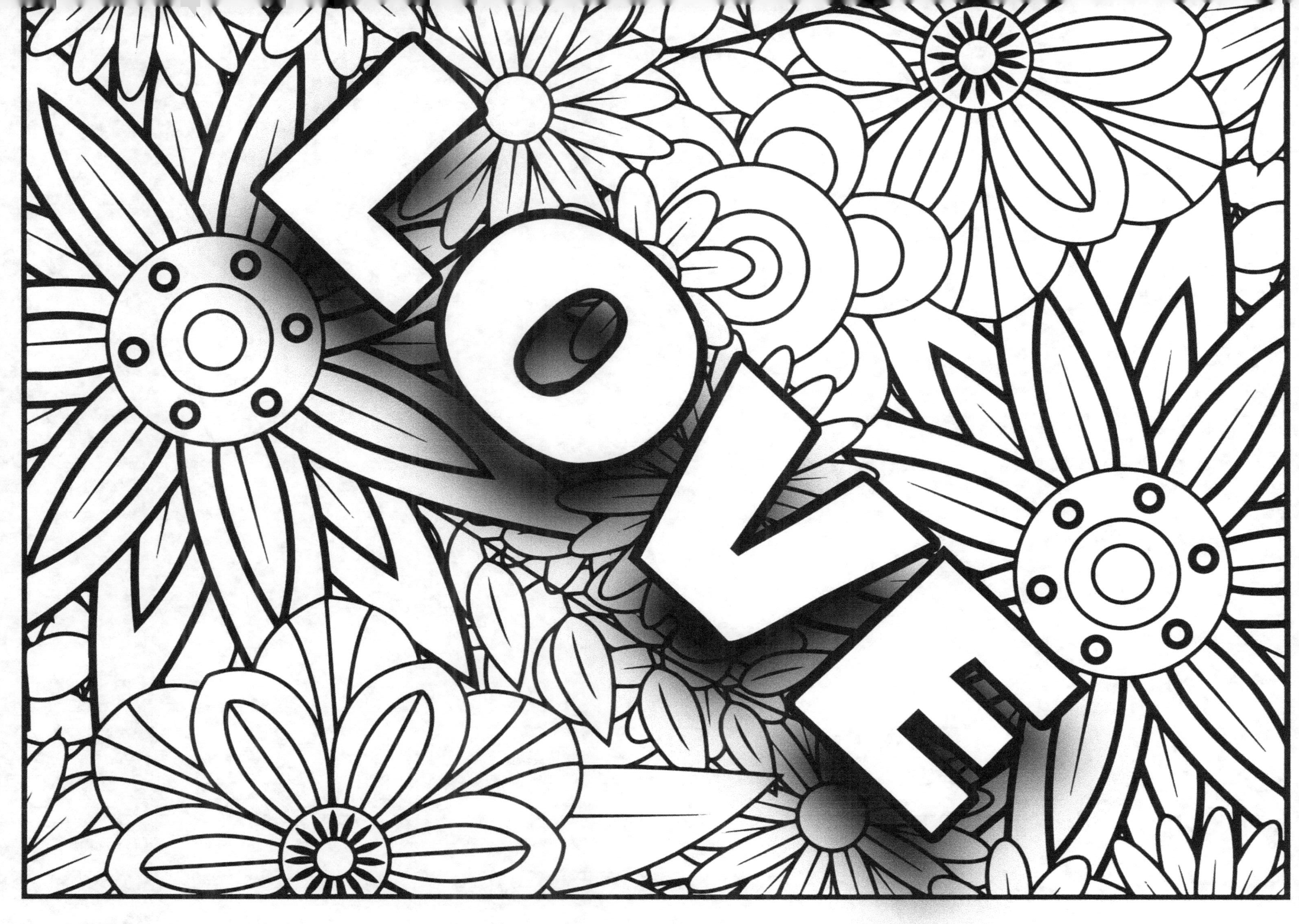
LOVE